RHINOPLASTY

Edited by **Michael J. Brenner**

Rhinoplasty
Edited by Michael J. Brenner

Published by InTech
Janeza Trdine 9, 51000 Rijeka, Croatia

Publishing Process Manager Sasa Leporic

Technical Editor Teodora Smiljanic

Cover Designer InTech Design Team

Additional hard copies can be obtained from orders@intechopen.com

Rhinoplasty, Edited by Michael J. Brenner
p. cm.
ISBN 978-953-307-849-6

For EU product safety concerns:
IN TECH d.o.o., Prolaz Marije Krucifikse Kozulić 3, 51000 Rijeka, Croatia,
info@intechopen.com or visit our website at intechopen.com.

Meet the editor

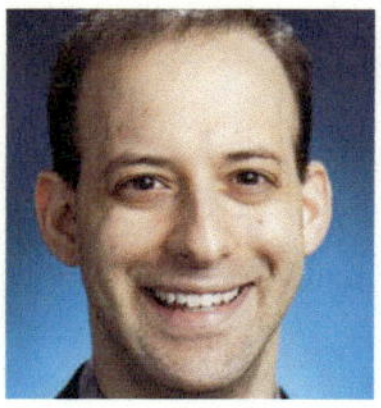

Dr. Michael J. Brenner, M.D., F.A.C.S is Director of Facial Plastic & Reconstructive Surgery at SIU School of Medicine. Dr Brenner was awarded his medical degree through the 7-year Honors Program in Medical Education at Northwestern University Medical School. He went on to perform residency in the 7-year Advanced Clinical Scholars Program in Otolaryngology – Head & Neck Surgery at Washington University Medical School, completing a two year Plastic Surgery Research Fellowship. His training culminated with a fellowship in Facial Plastic & Reconstructive Surgery at University of Minnesota and he now directs the facial plastic surgery program. Dr Brenner holds leadership positions in the American Academy for Facial Plastic & Reconstructive Surgery and is a delegate for the American Medical Association. He has also received several national distinctions for his pioneering research on nerve regeneration. He has lectured extensively, and has authored over 50 articles and book chapters in the field of facial plastic surgery. Dr Brenner specializes in rhinoplasty and also performs the full spectrum of cosmetic and reconstruction procedures, including cosmetic facelift surgery, blepharoplasty, forehead and brow lift surgery, necklift, scar revision, otoplasty, and treatment of traumatic and cancer-related deformities of the face and neck, including microvascular free tissue transfer.

Contents

Preface

Rhinoplasty is one of the defining procedures of plastic and reconstructive surgery, and it retains its stature as the most diverse and challenging of all plastic surgery procedures. Its roots stem from early efforts in nasal reconstruction and contemporary rhinoplasty reflects a rich history dating back to early descriptions of forehead reconstruction thousands of years ago. The emergence of modern rhinoplasty as a nuanced restorative and artistic procedure has allowed for an evolution of surgical technique that continues to the present day. As the most central and prominent facial features, the nose has distinct anatomic features that render it uniquely susceptible to injury and to scrutiny. Success in rhinoplasty is predicated on an understanding of structural and aesthetic considerations. The art and science of nasal surgery is truly a marriage of form and function.

This book describes the most recent clinical and research perspectives in the field of rhinoplasty. The contributing authors reach across specialty and international borders, sharing ideas from their respective surgical fields; this work should have broad appeal to an international readership. Over the years, rhinoplasty has matured into a field that strikes a balance between structural correction and aesthetic refinement. Contemporary thinking on rhinoplasty emphasizes a balance between preservation of supporting structures and a wide variety of approaches to rebuilding natural contours and structure through judicious resection and grafting. Surgical methods are continuously refined and have been influenced by new approaches in tissue engineering. The advent of open access publishing has afforded an unprecedented opportunity for reaching rhinoplasty surgeons around the world with these vital clinical and research innovations.

This book begins with a discussion of the rudiments of nasal analysis and planning, discusses execution of surgical techniques, and concludes with consideration of surgical complications. Opening chapters by Dr's Pawel Szychta and Abdullah Etoz cover preoperative assessment of the rhinoplasty patient, anthropometric analysis of the nose, and ethnic aspects of nasal anatomy. Dr Rui Xavier details experience with a modified delivery approach that improves precision and preservation of support in endonasal rhinoplasty. Dr Norifumi Nakamura elaborates on an elegant conceptual and practical approach to correction of unilateral and bilateral cleft lip nasal deformity. Dr Salvador Rodríguez-Camps Devís describes long term outcomes in combining temporalis fascia grafting with alar resection in tip rhinoplasty. Dr Paul O'Keeffe details progress in the use of a thin Medpor nasal shell for reconstituting nasal structure, and Dr. Aleksandar Vlahovic provides background and practical surgical approach to the challenging area of nasal hemangiomas. Closing chapters by Dr Sarit Cohen and Aris Ntomouchtsis consider minimally invasive approaches and mucous cysts as a complication of rhinoplasty.

This unique book thus provides invited treatises on the breadth of rhinoplasty from a diverse set of leaders in the field. The contributors collectively present expertise from the fields of plastic and reconstructive surgery, facial plastic surgery, and oral-maxillofacial surgery. Their collective experience as thought leaders covers a broad swath of cosmetic and reconstructive rhinoplasty specialists. Included herein are critical analytic insights, a wealth of illustrations, and accompanying schematics and clinical photographs. This volume serves as a resource for both students and for experienced aesthetic and reconstructive surgeons wishing to expand their understanding of rhinoplasty. Within this book is a wealth of proven and innovative approaches ranging from minor refinement to major reconstruction. The diversity of subjects covered reflects the inherent complexity of the art and science of rhinoplasty.

In tracing the development of rhinoplasty from early reconstructive efforts to the sophisticated aesthetic and restorative techniques of modern day, one can appreciate the rich history of this specialty. Within this volume are philosophies and approaches intended to provide a balanced perspective on the ever changing field of rhinoplasty. Discussion of structural grafting and approaches to augmentation are counterbalanced by consideration of judicious resection and refinement. Correction of congenital deformities is followed by consideration of acquired complications. The overarching goal of this work is to instill an understanding of the subtleties of nasal structure and how nasal anatomy can be adapted to maximize function and achieve a natural, pleasing appearance. The dedicated rhinoplasty surgeon progressively grows in his or her understanding of nasal anatomy, developing an armamentarium of skills over the course of many years of dutiful study. It is the purpose of this book to serve the reader as a trusted companion in this journey.

Michael J. Brenner
Southern Illinois University School of Medicine
USA

Part 1

Nasal Analysis

1

Anthropometric Analysis of the Nose

Abdullah Etöz
Aesthetic, Plastic and Reconstructive Surgery, Bursa
Turkey

1. Introduction

Anthropometric analysis is a method, aiming to achieve the most reliable comparison of the body forms by using specific landmarks determined in respect of anatomical prominences. Owing to the previous anthropometric studies, it is getting easier to discuss about the differences in between the ethnic and racial groups, and to compare the individual variations in both sexes. A great body of work in craniofacial anthropometry is that of Farkas who established a database of anthropometric norms by measuring and comparing more than 100 dimensions (linear, angular and surface contour's) (DeCarlo, 1998).

Today, anthropometric methods and surgical practice intersected at the point to treat congenital or post-traumatic facial disfigurements in various racial or ethnic groups successfully (Farkas et al 2005). The nose is a person's most defining feature because it is at the center of the face. The shape of the nose is a signature indicating the ethnicity, race, age and sex (Ofodile, 1995; Milgrim et al 1996; Mishima et al 2002; Ochi, 2002; Romo, 2003; Ferrario et al 1997; Bozkir et al 2004; Leong, 2004; Uzun et al 2006). Nasoplasty surgeons require access to facial databases based on accurate anthropometric measurements to perform optimum correction in both sexes.

There are several anthropometric studies related with the nose, which are bringing forward other different methods. However we decide to review a landmark-based geometric morphometric technique which can be easily used to analyze the nasal shapes in any population.

The shape differences in nasal anatomy between male and female are important thus, feminization of a male nose is an undesirable result. A successful outcome in rhinoplasty requires a thorough and accurate preoperative planning, and awareness of the morphological differences. Anthropometric analysis of nose is showing us a way to provide data which should contribute to satisfactory results of the cosmetic nasal surgery.

List of abbreviations used in the manuscript:

NHP: Natural head position

EDMA: Euclidean Distance Matrix Analysis

2. Anthropometric measurements

Anthropometric analysis of nasal anatomy is based on the comparison of measurements which are obtained separately from the anterior, lateral and inferior aspects. These measurements can be performed both by direct and indirect methods. Direct methods are

time-consuming and have several other disadvantages such as difficulty of patient adaptation (especially in children and infants), problems concerning repeatability of measurements and archiving of data. Therefore, indirect measurement methods including photograph, cephalogram, stereophotograph, laser scanning, and computerized tomography have increasingly become popular in recent years. The most frequent methods used clinically are photogrammetry and cephalometry. Photogrammetry is a fast and inexpensive method with superior patient compliance. The most important disadvantage of two-dimensional photogrammetry is its inability to assess facial depth. Three-dimensional photogrammetry appears to be a more appropriate technique in this respect.
The following issues are crucial in anthropometric analysis of the nose:

1. Standardization of the method
2. Landmark identification

2.1 Standardization of the method

Details of standardization of the methods used in anthropometric analysis have previously been defined by several investigators and are beyond the scope of this review. It is important to note that a standard head position is essential for any facial measurement. Natural head position (NHP) is the most appropriate since it is the most reproducible and provides a natural face orientation for treatment planning.

2.2 Landmark identification

The accurate identification and reliability of the landmarks are the most important indicators of the accuracy of the anthropometric measurements. One way to increase accuracy is to mark the landmarks before measuring. Many soft tissue landmarks reflect underlying bony structure. The bony points must be palpated with a finger to find the soft tissue equivalent. While some soft tissue points can be marked with a dermographic pen, some soft tissue landmarks such as endocanthion, exocanthion, cheilion, and crista philtre can be clearly identified without palpation. In photogrammetry, meticulous identification of soft tissue landmarks and marking of the landmarks determined by inspection and palpation before the acquisition of photographs will certainly improve the reliability of measurements. Nasal landmarks are presented in Figure-1 and Table 1.

1-2: al, Alare, the point where the nasal blade (ala nasi) extends farthest out
3: sn, Subnasale, the midpoint of the columella base
4-5: c′, Columella apex, the most anterior, or the highest point on the columella crest at the apex of the nostril
6: prn, Pronasale, the most prominent point on the nasal tip
*** 7-8:** The estimated junction of upper and lower lateral cartilages
9-10: mf, Maxilloanteriorale, where the maxilloanterioral and nasoanterioral sutures meet
11: n, Nasion, the point in the midline of both the anatomic nose and the nasoanterioral suture

Table 1. Anthropometric landmarks of nose from the anterior aspect. The numbers, abbreviations and definitions of the examined landmarks. The constructed landmarks are indicated by "*" sign

* **1:** the junction of nasolabial crease and nasal blade (ala nasi) **2: prn, Pronasale,** the most prominent point on the nasal tip **3: sn, Subnasale,** the midpoint of the columella base **4**: **al, Alare**, the point where the nasal blade (ala nasi) extends farthest out * **5:** the most prominent point of medial cruris of alar cartilage * **6:** the most prominent point of lateral cruris of alar cartilage 7: **c′, Columella apex,** the most anterior, or the highest point on the columella crest at the apex of the nostril * **8**: The ending point of the nasolabial fold * **9:** The estimated junction of nasal and maxillary bones * **10:** The most prominent point of nasal dorsum (nasal hump) * **11:** The estimated insertion point of medial cantus 12: **n, Nasion,** the point in the midline of both the anatomic nose and the nasoanterioral suture

Table 2. Anthropometric landmarks of nose from the lateral aspect. The numbers, abbreviations and definitions of the examined landmarks. The constructed landmarks are indicated by "*" sign

1-2: al, Alare, the point where the nasal blade (ala nasi) extends farthest out **3: sn, Subnasale,** the midpoint of the columella base * **4-5:** The most convex point of lateral cruris of alar cartilage **6: prn, Pronasale,** the most prominent point on the nasal tip

Table 3. Anthropometric landmarks of nose from the inferior aspect. The numbers, abbreviations and definitions of the examined landmarks. The constructed landmarks are indicated by "*" sign

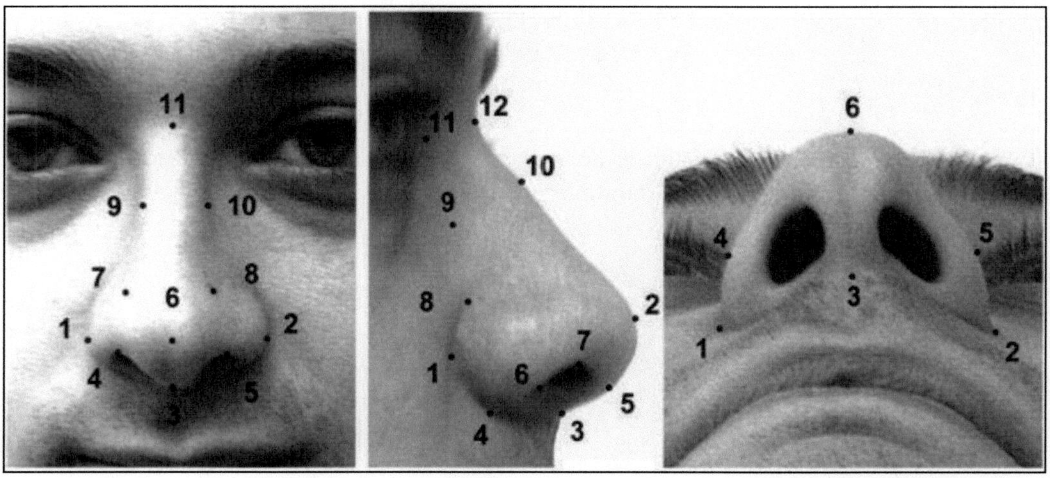

Fig. 1. Anthropometric (anterior 1-6, 9-11; lateral 2-4 and 12; inferior 1-3, 6) and constructed (anterior 7, 8; lateral 1, 5-11; inferior 4, 5) landmarks which were used in the anthropometric analysis of the nose

Key Point:
Photogrammetry is an easier and more effective method for anthropometric analysis of the nose.

	Anterior Aspect	Lateral Aspect	Inferior Aspect
The greater interlandmark distances in males (P < 0.05)	2Y6, 7Y8, 2Y7, 1Y3, 1Y6, 2Y3, 1Y8, 4Y5, 1Y5, 2Y4, 9Y10, 1Y2	4Y10, 6Y10, 8Y10, 7Y9, 3Y9, 5Y11, 5Y12, 3Y10, 7Y10, 2Y11, 4Y6, 2Y12, 3Y5, 4Y7, 5Y10, 5Y9, 6Y7, 2Y4, 6Y8, 2Y9, 2Y10, 2Y6, 2Y7, 3Y8, 1Y2, 7Y8, 9Y10, 4Y5, 1Y7, 2Y8, 1Y6, 5Y8, 1Y5, 3Y6, 5Y6, 1Y4, 3Y4, 1Y3, 5Y7,	2Y3, 3Y5, 3Y4, 2Y4, 1Y3, 1Y2, 1Y5, 4Y5
The greater interlandmark distances in females (P < 0.05)	4Y9, 3Y9, 1Y9, 2Y10, 6Y9, 5Y10, 3Y10, 6Y10, 7Y9, 3Y11, 6Y11, 8Y10, 4Y11, 5Y11, 4Y7, 5Y8	1Y9, 1Y11, 8Y9,	3Y6, 2Y5, 2Y6, 1Y6, 1Y4

Table 4. The Inter-landmark Distances Found to be Significantly Different Between Males and Females. In figure 2 these interlandmark distances were shown by bold and thin lines

Total length of nasal bridge	(n-prn)
Morphological width of nose	(al-al)
Nasal root width	(mf-mf)
Anatomical width of nose	(ac-ac)
Tip protrusion	(prn-sn)

Table 5. The common names for interlanmark distances of the nose

	Males		Females	
	r	p	r	p
MorphologicNasal Width / Nasal Root Width	.616	<0.001	.345	0.001
MorphologicNasal Width / Length of nasal bridge	.651	<0.001	.409	<0.001
Morphologic Nasal Width / Anatomical width of nose	.612	<0.001	.317	0.003
MorphologicNasal Width / Tip protrusion	.299	0.007	.286	0.008
Nasal Root Width / Length of nasal bridge	.492	<0.001	.439	<0.001
Nasal Root Width / Anatomical width of nose	.392	<0.001	-	p>0.05
Nasal Root Width / Tip protrusion	.351	0.001	-	p>0.05
Length of nasal bridge / Anatomical width of nose	.410	<0.001	.223	0.039
Length of nasal bridge / Tip protrusion	.405	<0.001	.378	<0.001
Anatomical width of nose/ Tip protrusion	.527	<0.001	.761	<0.001

Table 6. For example, the data showing us the statistical correlations of the interlandmark distances of nose in both sex

Landmark reliability

It is important to understand the various sources of error that can affect anthropometric measurements during location of landmarks. Lack of precision results in variability among repeated measurements of the same specimen and has two components:

- Observer error in locating landmarks
- Instrument error in identifying landmark coordinates (Lele, 1991 and 1993).

It is crucial to analyze the reliability of the landmarks. Optimal standard to achieve reliability is that all landmarks should be marked by the same investigator on all subjects. Instrumental errors should be avoided by using a standardized digital photographic imaging taken from anterior, lateral and inferior aspects by using a constantly stable digital camera (Hwang, 2003; Uzun et al 2006).

Collection of two-dimensional craniofacial landmarks of nose

The data collection procedure should take place in two separate steps, and followed by off-line calculations. At first, for each subject, digital photographic images should be taken by the same investigator using an at least 2.0 mega pixel digital camera. At the second stage, the examined landmarks are marked on these digital images. Anthropometric landmarks are defined in Figure-1. The landmarks shown in the figure are also accepted in previous anthropometric studies (Farkas et al 1998). For enrichment of nasal anthropometric analysis, some "constructed" landmarks are also used. These landmarks are determined by constructing a line tangent to another landmark or a bony edge. The descriptions of the examined landmarks are done in Table 1 and shown in Figure 1.

For each subject, eleven landmarks (five anthropometric and two constructed) in the anterior aspect, twelve landmarks (four anthropometric and eight constructed) in the lateral aspect and six landmarks (four anthropometric and two constructed) in the inferior aspect of nose are defined. The landmarks were marked on the digital photographs by using TPSDIG 2.04 software. This software was developed by F. James Rohlf and it is one of the most frequently used software both for the marking the landmarks (however, what is recommended is to take photos after marking the landmarks on the person) and for determining the inter-landmark distances in pixels. A ruler is used in the shooting for the measurement of the distances between the landmarks in digital images and later on the unit distance (1 cm) is calibrated with its equivalent in pixel in order to obtain measurement values separately.

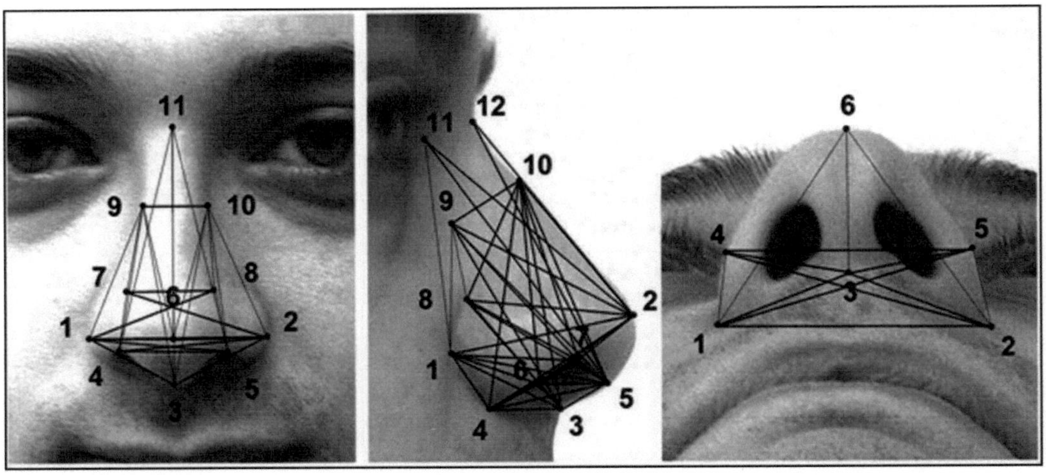

Fig. 2. The inter-landmark distances, viewed from anterior, lateral and inferior aspects. These distances could be measured by computer scales in photogrammetric computer programs and the results should be proportionate to each other. For example in this figure, the *thin lines* indicate the inter-landmark distances which were found to be greater in females; the *bold lines* indicate the inter-landmark distances which were found to be greater in males

It was proven to be reliable in studies including facial landmarks by Nechala (1999) and Ferrario et al (2003) which compared photogrammetry with direct measurements, and showed that sharp facial profile contours could eliminate the differences between the direct and indirect measurements of the nose. The strengths and limitations of photogrammetry must be appreciated. However, it is ideally suited to the evaluation of proportions, as the magnification factor is eliminated (Weigberg, 2005).

Statistical studies of anatomical shape variations in population are important in understanding anatomical effects of diseases or biological processes. Several procedures for obtaining shape information from landmark data have been proposed. Euclidean Distance Matrix Analysis (EDMA) is used to calculate all possible linear distances among landmarks by creating matrixes for each subject. EDMA results are actually related to the coordinate-system-invariant properties that make EDMA biologically and statistically advantageous (Theodore, 1998).

Ethnic influences can result in different appearances of the nose, as follows: Caucasian, leptorrhine; African American, platyrrhine; Hispanic, paraleptorrhine; and Asian, subplatyrrine. For example, there are three types of African American noses are described:

African, Afro-Caucasian, and Afro-Indian (Ofodile, 1995). There are also variations of nasal shape related to sex in both ethnic groups. Nose shape gives information about race, ethnicity, age and sex. The size, shape, and proportions of the nose provide a visual basis suggesting the character of the person. Moreover, it is an important key for a natural and aesthetically pleasing human face (Aung et al, 2000). Accordingly, concern about the nasal shape has recently increased; lots of people want to have rhinoplasty operations. Any surgeon who performs rhinoplasty must be keenly aware of the morphological differences in nasal anatomy between male and female. The planning of the cosmetic nasal surgery must take into consideration psychological aspects, differences in skin conditions, and anthropometric measurements.

There have been many methods on the anatomic evaluation of the nose and variations in different racial and ethnic groups however there is an easy and reliable way to analysis nose shape: Photogrammetric nasal analysis which is based on framework and thought to be a better way to examine the differences of nose according to conventional methods.

3. Applications to other areas of health and disease

Today, the anthropometric methods and surgical practice intersected at a point to treat the congenital or post-traumatic facial disfigurements in various racial or ethnic groups successfully. Rhinoplasty surgeons require access to facial databases based on accurate anthropometric measurements to perform optimum correction in both sexes. There should be some points to be brought to mind during the cosmetic nasal surgery for men because of different expectations, which is not technically different from the one for women. Anthropometric analysis is a step to clarify these important points and basement for enhancing the plans of the corrective surgery.

4. Practical guidelines

- The subjects have to be recruited from a population who has no noticeable nasal, facial disfigurement and no history of previous nasal or facial surgery .
- Demographic data obtained included age, place of birth, and parental heritage.
- The subjects are rested for 10 minutes before the photography.
- A constant, stable three-leg camera holder is used and all the subjects are positioned at the same distance from the camera.
- All data was obtained from standardized digital photographic images taken from anterior, lateral and inferior aspects by using a digital camera.
- Anthropometric landmarks were defined regarding a previous report of Farkas et al.
- For enrichment of shape analysis, some "constructed" landmarks can be used, meaning that the definition of the landmark is determined by constructing a line to another landmark or bony edge.
- The landmarks should be marked by the same investigator on the digital photographs by using a digital imaging software.

5. Summary points

- Statistical studies of anatomical shape variations in population are important in understanding anatomical effects of diseases or biological processes.

- Anthropometric analysis of facial asymmetry is based on the comparison of homolog measurements that are obtained separately from the anterior, lateral and inferior aspects.
- Standardization of method, accurate identification of landmarks to be used in the measurements in nasal anthropometric analysis.
- Anthropometric analysis is a step to clarify these important points and basement for enhancing the plans of the corrective surgery.

6. References

Aung S.C. (2000) Br J Plast Surg 53: 109–116
Bozkir M.G. (2004) Surg Radiol Anat 26:212-219
DeCarlo D. (1998) An Anthropometric face model using variational techniques. 25th Annual Conference on Computer Graphics and Interactive Techniques. Appeared in Proceedings SIGGRAPH' 98, pp 67-74
Farkas L.G. (2005) J Craniofacial Surg 16: 615-646
Ferrario V.F. (1997) Cleft Palate Craniofac J 34:309-317
Ferrario V.F. (2003) Clin Anat 16:420-443
Hwang T-S, Kang H-S. (2003) Ann Anat 185:189-193
Lele S, Richtsmeier J.T. (1991) Am J Phys Anthropol 86:415–428
Lele S (1993) Math. Geol. 25:573–602
Leong S.C.L., White P.S. (2004) Clin Otolaryngol 29:672-676
Milgrim L.M. (1996) Arch Otolaryngol Head Neck Surg 122:1079-1086
Mishima K. (2002) Cell Tissues Organs 170: 198-206
Nechala P. (1999) Plast Reconstr Surg 103:1819-1825
Ochi K, Ohashi T (2002) Otolaryngol Head Neck Surg 126:160-163
Ofodile F.A., Bokhari F (1995) Ann Plast Surg 34:123-129
Romo T, Abraham M.T. (2003) Fac Plast Surg 19:269-277
Rohlf FJ. http://life.bio.sunysb.edu/ee/rohlf/software.html
Theodore M.C. III, Richtsmeier J.T. (1998) Am J Phys Anthropol 107:273–283
Uzun A. (2006) Auris Nasus Larynx 33:31-35
Weinberg S.M., Kolar J.C. (2005) J Craniofac Surg 16(5):847-51

2

Preoperative Planning for Rhinoplasty, in Relation to the Gender and Ethnicity

Pawel Szychta[1,2], Ken J. Stewart[2] and Jan Rykala[2]
[1]*Plastic and Reconstructive Surgery Department, St John's Hospital, Livingston*
[2]*Plastic, Reconstructive and Aesthetic Surgery Department, 1st University Hospital, Lodz*
[1]*Great Britain*
[2]*Poland*

1. Introduction

The nose plays an important role in the respiratory tract and is one of the most visible organs on the face due to its central position. It emphasizes the shape of the eyes, is an integral part of the face, and co-decides for its aesthetics as a whole. In clinical practice, there is no universal concept of the 'perfect face', nor is there a specific shape of the nose, considered a model of beauty. Normal range of the values describing nasal shape varies depending on race and gender. In order to achieve a very good result of aesthetic surgery for an each individual patient, surgeon must include to the preoperative planning of rhinoplasty the differences of nasal shape in relation to gender and ethnicity.

2. Anthropometry for individual analysis of the nasal shape

Precise preoperative planning is essential in obtaining good results after rhinoplasty, judged subjectively by the patient and surgeon. Anthropometric measurements of the nose can be helpful in preoperative objective analysis. They serve both to highlight the parameters that require correction, as well as pointing to some of the correct proportions, which should be preserved during surgery (Szychta et al. 2010).

2.1 Devices for measuring the nasal shape

Until recently, anthropometric measurements were carried out directly on the patient using rulers and anthropometric calipers or indirectly on standardized photographs. These methods cannot be used in routine clinical practice as they are time-consuming and inaccurate.

An innovative method for measuring the surface of the human body is three-dimensional imaging. It involves taking standardized pictures of the analyzed region using specialized equipment connected to the computer, and then analyzing the three-dimensional digital model. The advantages of this method include accuracy, speed and automation of the calculations. Analysis with a 3D scanner was developed with relevant analytical software by one of the authors adds an additional 2 minutes to the time spent with patient (Szychta et al, 2010a). The invested time is minimal, taking into account the possibility of obtaining relevant, objective clinical data that may provide significant help in planning rhinoplasty. Reliability of measurements with a 3D scanner using the anatomical points has already been confirmed in the previous studies. The drawbacks of the currently available 3D scanners are their high, one-time cost and very low availability of the equipment adapted for clinical use.

2.2 Outline of the analytical method of the nasal shape assessment

The authors propose an algorithm including linear measurements, angles and indices, which allow to depict the differences among people of both sexes and of different races (Szychta et al, 2010b). Assessment is based on 18 anthropometric nasal points (7 separate for left and right side of the body), including points describing the nostrils: anterior (naL, naR), posterior (npL, npR), lateral (nlL, nlR) and medial (nmL, nmR), as well as subalare (sbalL, sbalR) and alare (alL, alR), and also 7 single points of the nose: pronasale (prn), subnasale (sn), nasion (n), glabella (gl), rhinion (rh), labiale superius (ls) and columellar point (cp) (Figure 1).

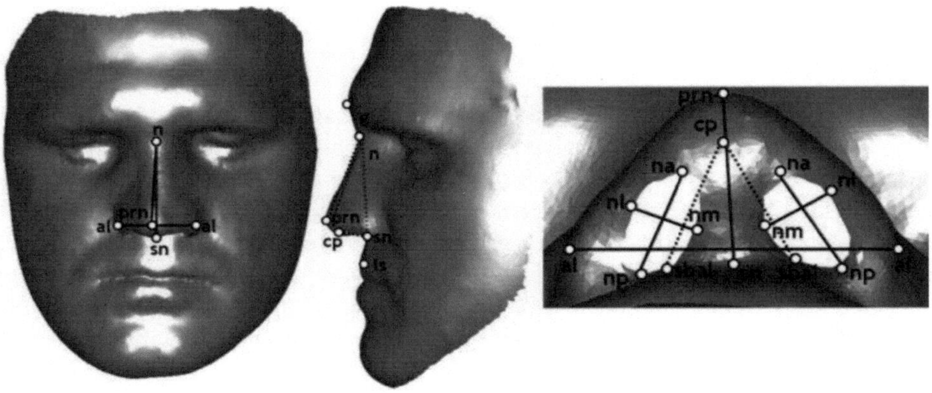

Fig. 1. Anatomical points used in the study together with indices of proportions (solid lines) and angles (dashed lines), shown on a sample three-dimensional model of the face in a patient after posttraumatic rhinoplasty. Views: a) front, b) profile, c) from below

By using selected anatomical points, the following 8 linear measurements are carried out: length and width for both nostrils (naR-npR, naL-npL, nlR-nmR and nlL-nmL, respectively), nasal height (n-sn), nasal length (n-prn), nasal width (al-al) and the nasal prominence (sn-prn). On the basis of linear measurements, two ratios of nasal proportions are determined: index of the prominence to the nasal width (sn-prn/al-al * 100) and nasal index (al-al/n-sn * 100).
The survey consists of 4 angles defining the shape of the nose: interaxial (sbalR-cp-sbalL), nasofrontal (gl-n-prn), nasolabial (cp-sn-ls) and nasofacial (prn-n-sn).

3. Ethnic differences in parameters describing facial and nasal shape

The aesthetic beauty of a nose is subjective and varies according to specific cultural and ethnic population (Table 1). A characteristics of the proper nasal shape depends on the race: the Caucasian nose (called leptorrhine - 'long and narrow'), the African nose (platyrrhine - 'a wide and flat') and the Asian nose (called mesorrhine – 'borderline') (Krzeski, 2005).
The Caucasian nose is characteristic of people of European descent, and its features are often used as a model for comparison with other races. The Caucasian nose is narrower than the

African and the Asian. It is also longer compared with other ethnic groups. Caucasians also have larger nostrils, compared with those of Mongoidal race (Table 1) (Rohrich & Bolden, 2010).

Parameter of the nose		Sex	Our study, (Caucasian race) n=54		Caucasian race (Farkas, 1994a), n=50		Caucasian race (Leong et al., 2006), n=50		Negroid race (Ofodile & Bokhari, 1995), n=69		Mongoloid race: Chinese (Farkas et al., 1994b), n=60		Mongoloid race: Singaporeans (Aung et al., 1995), n=90		Mongoloid race: Koreans (Hwang & Kang, 2003), n=265	
			mean	SD	mean	SD	mean	SD	mean	SD	mean	SD	mean	SD	mean	SD
Width (mm)		F	32.15	3.73	31.40	1.90	36		40.00	0.4	37.20	2.10	37.63	3.47	37.2	2.3
		M	34.89	4.35	34.70	2.60	36		43.50	0.39	39.20	2.90	39.49	2.95	40.7	2.4
Height (mm)		F	55.81	4.36	48.90	2.60			49.30	0.42	51.70	2.30	46.93	3.30		
		M	60.02	4.23	53.00	3.50			52.40	0.44	53.50	2.80	50.15	4.16		
Length (mm)		F	45.66	5.58							44.30	3.70	40.04	3.62		
		M	49.02	6.60							46.20	2.80	43.65	4.50		
Prominence (mm)		F	19.29	3.96	19.30	1.90			20.40	0.32	15.40	1.80	16.69	2.01	20.2	1.9
		M	20.66	2.95	20.60	2.20			23.10	0.36	16.10	1.50	17.68	1.66	21.7	1.8
Right nostril	Width (mm)	F	9.63	1.96											6	1
		M	10.47	2.09											6.6	1.1
	Length (mm)	F	15.61	2.14											10.8	1.2
		M	16.25	1.92											12	1.4
Left nostril	Width (mm)	F	9.49	1.81											6	1
		M	10.25	1.94											6.5	1.1
	Length (mm)	F	15.92	2.48											10.8	1.2
		M	16.71	1.93											12.1	1.4
Nasofrontal angle (°)		F	132.95	5.99	134	7.40	137.5	4.8	131.9	6.8	135.6	4.40	139.09	7.65		
		M	131.05	5.10	130.5	8.10	129.3	12.1	135.6	5.4	134.5	7.00	137.43	8.10		
Nasolabial angle (°)		F	104.23	11.21	99.1	8.70	101.1	8.6	91	9.3	88.5	11.20	97.71	12.65		
		M	103.67	10.31	98.9	8.00	95.6	10.2	83.5	10.5	86.9	12.20	99.91	7.39		
Interaxial angle (°)		F	69.02	11.89									80.67	10.96	76.9	18.3
		M	66.32	13.21									75.07	10.65	84.8	24.5
Nasofacial angle (°)		F	33.06	4.16			37.2	5.4								
		M	31.64	3.01			36.7	7.8								
Nasal index (%)		F	57.72	5.93	64.21				81.70				79	7.00		
		M	58.25	6.92	64.85				83.80				81	9.00		
Index of prominence to width (%)		F	60.49	13.95	61.46				51.5				45	6.00	53.9	5.6
		M	59.56	7.89	59.36				53.8				45.77	4.00	52.9	5.8

Table 1. Parameters describing the shape of the nose in relation to gender in healthy white, black and Asian race, compared with our results of rhinoplasty in group of Europeans (Szychta et al. 2011)

The African nose is characterized by a wide base, short and concave bridge and nasofrontal angle of 130-140 degrees. It is said to be pear-shape. Relatively short tip projection is often encountered, as well as posteriorly extended alae and round nostrils. Very thick skin of the nose is observed. Black people have the widest and most prominent nose compared with other ethnic groups. Within Europe of course interracial nasal differences are recognized by all (Patrocinio LG & Patrocinio JA, 2007).
The Asian nose has intermediate characteristics between representatives of Caucasian and African. The skin of the nose is quite thick and the bridge is wide. Analyzing cartilaginous-osseous skeleton, nasal bones are usually short. Nasal tip is rounded off with an insufficient projection, rotation and recessed columella. Typically, the nostrils are slightly rounded. The shape of the nose is similar in representatives of the Mongoidal race: Chinese, Singaporeans and Koreans, with clearly more prominent nose in the last group (Table 1) (Farkas et al., 1994b; Aung et al., 1995; Hwang & Kang, 2003; Lam, 2009).
Additionally, patients can sometimes seek to conform to culturally accepted perceptions of an attractive nose. For example, Black or Asian patients living in predominantly Caucasian societies not uncommonly seek surgery to enhance nasal projection (Niechajev & Haraldsson, 1997).

4. Differences in normal values of the nasal shape in relation to gender

The range of values of the anthropometric parameters defining the 'ideal aesthetic face' and 'ideal aesthetic nose' is different for male and female (Table 2). These differences must be

Anatomic nasal parameter	Anthropometric nasal parameter	Women	Men
Height	Height	Smaller	Larger
Dorsum width	Nasal index	Narrower	Wider
Alae width	Nasal width	Narrower	Wider
Nostrils	Length and width of both nostrils	Smaller	Larger
Projection	Fronto-nasal angle, Naso-facial angle	Smaller	Larger
Nasal tip	Naso-labial angle	More cranial rotation	More caudal rotation
Nasal root	Nasion-glabella lenght	Superior eyelid crease or just below	Superior eyelid crease or just above
Line of the nasal dorsum	Angle of deviation between cartilaginous and osseous vault	Straight or a bit concave; acceptable small depression of the nasal dorsum	Straight or a bit convex; acceptable small nasal hump
Soft tissues layer		Thinner	Thicker

Table 2. Overall, comparative characteristics of the normal nasal shape in women and men (Krzeski, 2005)

taken into account when planning the surgery. During each preoperative evaluation of the nose, the proportions of the nose must create harmony with the rest of the individual face. It is commonly held view that women have larger eyes, smaller noses, fuller lips, a smaller distance between lips and chin, a smaller lower lip and a gently outlined maxilla. In contrast, an attractive man has close and deep placement of eyes, bigger nose, pronounced cheekbones and jaw, as well as clearly outlined non-prominent ears (Gunter et al., 2007).
Rhinoplasty techniques for men and women are identical, differing only within the scope of the resection. Lack of understanding of differences in the shape of the nose in relation to gender may lead to adverse aesthetic outcome (e.g. feminization of the male nose), which is not a rare complication of rhinoplasty.

4.1 Our study

The authors examined the usefulness of the proposed method of anthropometric assessment of the nose, evaluating 43 patients treated in the Plastic, Reconstructive and Aesthetic Surgery Department (Medical University of Lodz, Poland) (33 men and 10 women) aged 18 to 45 years (mean 27 years) for the aesthetic results of posttraumatic rhinoplasty (Szychta et al. 2011). The results were compared with previously described values of anthropometric parameters for the healthy population. In order to standardize the study group, only Caucasians of both genders have been included to the research. All patients underwent partial resection and reposition of the nasal septum, placing it in the median plane of the body. Simultaneously, the osteotomy of the nasal skeleton was performed. Three-dimensional images using 3D scanner were performed at 6 months after surgery. Subsequently, the anthropometric measurements of the three-dimensional facial model were carried out with a computer program. Linear measurements were performed with an accuracy of about 0.1 millimeter.
The shape of the nose in men and women showed significant differences (Table 1). According to the results obtained in previous studies, women had narrower and shorter nose (width: 32.15 ± 3.73 mm and 34.89 ± 4.35 mm, height: 55.81 ± 4.36mm and 60.02 ± 4.23mm, respectively). In women, the nostrils were rounder, with similar width and shorter length in comparison to men (width of the nostrils: $p > 0.05$, length of the right and left nostril: $p = 0.0457$, $p = 0.0207$, respectively). For both sexes we observed the same ratio between width and height of the nose as well as between its prominence and width. We did not notice differences in the position of the nasal tip in relation to the whole face.
In conclusion, the nose was usually smaller in women. We obtained good results of rhinoplasty, which were similar to healthy Caucasian population in majority of the linear parameters. However, the nasal index was lower compared with the control group due to the surgical narrowing of nasal tip. Moreover, in the present study, slightly more obtuse nasolabial angle than in the healthy population was associated with the surgical shortening of the nasal tip. Increased nasofrontal angle and the associated reduced nasofacial angle versus the comparison group resulted from osteotomy and the related shift of the nasal root (nasion).
Further studies are planned to determine whether the introduction of the presented method to clinical practice improves the aesthetic outcome of rhinoplasty. The comparative assessment of pre- and postoperative results after posttraumatic rhinoplasty with use of 3D scanner has been reported elsewhere (Szychta et al. 2010).

5. The individual aspect of rhinoplasty

Individualized nasal analysis should into account normative values based on patient's gender and race, as well as consideration of the individual shape of the face. The nose is an integral part of the face and must be adjusted in size and shape to the whole. Therefore, it is essential to obtain harmony between the parameters of the nose during posttraumatic rhinoplasty (Gunter et al., 2007). Even in healthy people with an aesthetically attractive appearance of the face, a number of parameters differ from the usual aesthetic standards. A long or oval face looks attractive with a longer and narrower nose. Similarly, a round or square face is more harmonious with the shorter and broader nose (Figure 2). During the preoperative assessment the surgeon should show understanding for the individual nasal proportions for each patient, treating the so called 'aesthetic proportions' only as a guideline and not seeking to achieve standard 'aesthetic ideal' (Tebbetts, 2008).

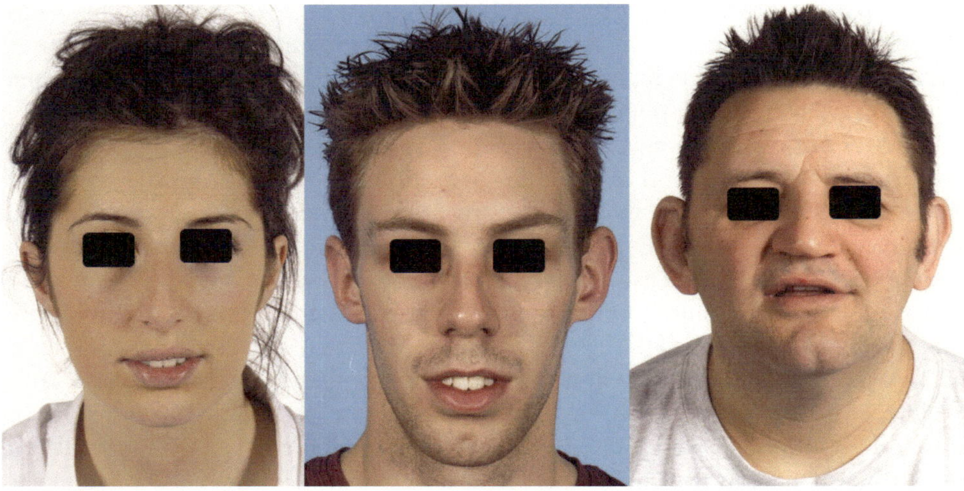

Fig. 2. Differently shaped faces with harmonious noses; a) and b) long face with long thin nose, c) round face with harmonious short, wide nose

Almost every human face among the healthy population has a significant asymmetry between the two sides of the body. Asymmetrical shape of the face can be interesting. It is also important that before the posttraumatic rhinoplasty the surgeon supports the patient with information regarding risks of postoperative deviations from perfect symmetry (Tardy, 1997).

In our opinion, knowledge of the normal range of values of parameters for a given gender and ethnicity is important to better understand the general principles of the correct nasal shape, along with the desire to obtain a perfect postoperative result, individually tailored by the operation.

6. Conclusions

The aesthetic characteristic of the nasal shape in a healthy Caucasian population is significantly different compared with the noses of other races. In the preoperative planning and evaluation of treatment results, knowledge of anthropometric differences between people of different races and both sexes appears equally important as the individual differences in relation to the whole face. Following the above mentioned guidelines in the study, we achieved similar aesthetic results of posttraumatic rhinoplasty to the relevant population with normal parameter values of the nasal shape.

7. References

Aung, S.C.; Ngim, R.C.K. & Lee, S.T. (1995). Evaluation of the laser scanner as a surface measuring tool and its accuracy compared with direct facial anthropometric measurements. British Journal of Plastic Surgery, (December 1995), Vol.48, No.8, pp.551–558, ISSN 0007-1226

Farkas, L.G. (Ed.). (1994a). Anthropometry of the head and face in medicine, 2nd edn., Raven, ISBN-13 9780781701594, New York, USA

Farkas, L.G.,; Ngim, R.C.K & Lee, S.T. (1994b). Craniofacial norms in 6-, 12-, and 18-year-old Chinese subjects. In: Leslie, G. & Farkas, L.G. (Eds.). Anthropometry of the head and face, 2nd edn., Raven, ISBN-13 978-0781701594, New York, USA, pp.201–218

Gunter, J.P.; Rohrich, R.J. & Adams, W.P. (Eds.). (2007). Dallas Rhinoplasty - Nasal Surgery by the Masters, 2nd edn., Quality Medical Publishing Inc., ISBN-13 978-1-57626-223-8, St. Louis, USA

Hwang, T.S. & Kang, H.S. (2003). Morphometry of nasal bases and nostrils in Koreans. Annals of Anatomy, Vol.185, No.2, (April 2003), pp.189–193, ISSN 0940-9602

Krzeski, A. (Ed.). (2005). [Wyklady z chirurgii nosa]. In Polish. 1st ed., Via Medica, ISBN 83-89861-29-1, Gdansk, Poland

Lam, S.M. (2009). Asian rhinoplasty. Seminars in Plastic Surgery, Vol.23, No.3, (August 2009), pp.215-22, ISSN 1535-2188

Leong, S.C.L. & White, P.S. (2006). A comparison of aesthetic proportions between the healthy Caucasian nose and the aesthetic ideal. Journal of Plastic, Reconstrive and Aesthetic Surgery, Vol.59, No.3, (March 2006), pp.248–252, ISSN 1748-6815

Niechajev, I. & Haraldsson, P.O. (1997). Ethnic progile of patients undergoing aesthetic rhinoplasty in Stockholm. Aesthetic Plastic Surgery, Vol.21, No.3, (May-June 1997), pp.139-145, ISSN 0364-216X

Ofodile, F.A. & Bokhari, F. (1995). The African-American nose: part II. Annals of Plastic Surgery, Vol.34, No.2, (February 1995), pp.123–129, ISSN 0148-7043

Patrocinio, L.G.; Patrocinio, J.A. (2007). Open rhinoplasty for African-American noses. British Journal of Oral and Maxillofacial Surgery, Vol.45, No.7, (October 2007), pp.561-566, ISSN 0940-9602

Rohrich, R.J. & Bolden, K. (2010). Ethnic rhinoplasty. Clinics in Plastic Surgery, Vol.37, No.2, (April 2010), pp.352-370, ISSN 0094-1298

Szychta, P.; Rykala, J. & Kruk-Jeromin, J. (2010). Assessment of 3D scanner usefulness in aesthetic evaluation of posttraumatic rhinoplasty. The 33rd European Academy of Facial Plastic Surgery Meeting, (September 2010), Belek, Turkey

Szychta, P.; Rykala, J. & Kruk-Jeromin, J. (2011). Individual and ethnic aspects of preoperative planning for posttraumatic rhinoplasty. European Journal of Plastic Surgery, Vol.34, No.8, (August 2011), pp.245-249, ISSN 1435-0130

Tardy, M.E. (Ed.). (1997). Rhinoplasty - The Art and the Science, 1st edn., W.B. Saunders Co., ISBN 0-7216-8755-5, Philadelphia, USA

Tebbetts, J.B. (Ed.). (2008). Primary Rhinoplasty - Redefining the Logic and Techniques, 2nd edn., Mosby Elsevier Inc., ISBN 978-0-323-04111-9, Philadelphia, USA

3

Preoperative Assessment

Pawel Szychta[1,2], Ken J. Stewart[1] and Jan Rykala[2]
[1]*Plastic and Reconstructive Surgery Department, St John's Hospital, Livingston*
[2]*Plastic, Reconstructive and Aesthetic Surgery Department, 1st University Hospital, Lodz*
[1]*Great Britain*
[2]*Poland*

1. Introduction

Rhinoplasty offers a substantial customization of the parameters of the operated area in comparison with most cosmetic procedures. At the same time, the surgeon faces a challenging task of matching the complex shape of the nose to the rest of the face. The face is a three-dimensional structure of highly-integrated anatomical components, gently intersecting one another. Therefore, detailed preoperative planning, based on accurate knowledge of the construction of the nose, can significantly contribute to achieve pleasing result after rhinoplasty.

2. Nasal aesthetics

The nose occupies a central position on the face, dictating, to a large extent, general facial aesthetics. There is no single model of ideal proportions of the face, or nose. Moreover, a slight facial asymmetry is considered an attractive trait. In practice, therefore, the concept of the normal range should be used instead of determining the 'ideal' values of parameters describing the proportions of the face and nose.
The result of rhinoplasty should be an attractive nose, harmonious with the rest of the face and emphasizing the beauty of the eyes (Tardy, 1997). The most favourable evaluation of patient before rhinoplasty is based on the proportions of nose with the whole face.

2.1 Nose as an integral part of the face

Examination of the patient prior to rhinoplasty should include assessment of all the facial components as complementary elements. Knowledge of normal proportions allows for accurate detection of deviations from existing standards and precise targeting of surgical correction in the establishment of an aesthetic shape of the nose, which is proportionate to the rest of the face.
Leonardo da Vinci's facial model is split into three equal horizontal parts, bounded by the lines intersecting four topographic points: trichion (hairline in the midline), glabella, subnasale (nasal spine) and menton (lower edge of the chin) (Figure 1) (Gunter et al., 2007). The upper third is the least important in the estimation of the proportion of the nose and face. The nose is in the middle third of the face. The lower third of the face (between subnasale and menton) is further divided by a horizontal line intersecting the commissure of the lips (stomion) into two parts: 1/3 upper and 2/3 lower.

In addition, Powell and Humphreys divided face into 5 vertical areas of equal width, bounded by six vertical lines: both, a) and b) lines passing through the inner canthi, which includes the medial part of the face with nose, both, c) and d) lines crossing the lateral canthi, denoting the lateral edge of the neck, both, e) and f) lines through the most outwardly situated point of the pinna (Powell & Humphreys, 1984).

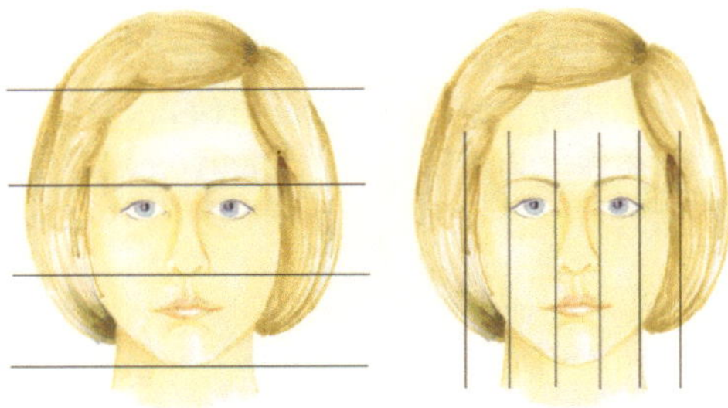

Fig. 1. a) Face divided into three equal horizontal parts by Leonardo da Vinci, b) face divided into 5 vertical areas of equal width

The correct proportions of the face vary depending on gender, race, and individual anatomical features. According to a beautiful face in relation to gender, attractive women have less marked jaw, bigger eyes and complementary smaller noses, as compared to men (Perrett et al., 1994). Aesthetically pleasing lips are fuller, with a smaller upper lip. Women also have a smaller distance between lips and chin. In contrast, men usually have a bigger nose than women, coupled with a deep placement of eyes, located close to each other. Attractive males have visible cheekbones and jaw. It is important that the ears in men are not prominent.

For educational purposes, the commonly used facial proportions relate to white women, who are the most common group of patients undergoing rhinoplasty (Talakoub & Wesley, 2009). It should be noted, however, that surgeons have to maintain the different relationships between the nose and face in individuals of both sexes and different races.

2.2 Nasal aesthetic subunits

The facial surface is divided into so-called aesthetic units, which are areas of skin with identical properties such as colour, texture, elasticity and thickness, and are often limited by the curvature of the surface of the body. They serve as guidelines for reconstruction in the event of loss of tissue. One of the units is the skin covering the nose. Its surface is divided into subunits, the knowledge of which can be helpful in understanding the nasal shape. There are nine aesthetic subunits of the nose: tip, columella, alar bases, alar side walls, dorsum and dorsal side walls (Figure 2) (Rahman et al., 2010). Any surgical incision placed between the subunits produces the least visible scars.

2.3 Characteristics of the correct shape of the nose

Preoperative evaluation is based largely on a conversation with a patient, observation of the nose and palpation. However, standardised photographs are a valuable addition in the preoperative analysis of the nasal shape, often highlighting the anatomical details, which are difficult to see during the examination. Regardless of the method of analysis, the surgeon should recognize the anatomical abnormalities of the nose, based on knowledge of the correct proportions of the face and nose. The characteristics of the aesthetic face and nose are described below.

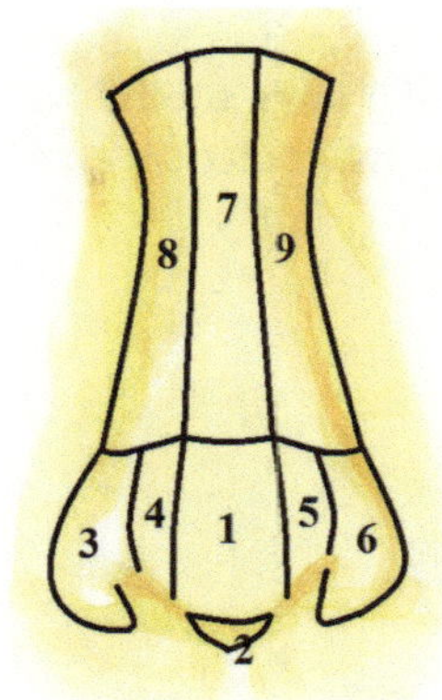

Fig. 2. Aesthetic subunits of the nose: 1 - tip subunit, 2 - columellar subunit, 3 and 6 - alar side wall subunits, 4 and 5 - alar base subunits, 7 - dorsal subunit, 8 and 9 - dorsal side wall subunits

From the anterior view (on examination/in the photograph), the nasal bridge changes gradually over its entire length, being narrowest in the area around the root (at the height of the medial supraorbital edge, nasion), while the broadest at the base (at the tip of the nose - pronasale) (Krzeski, 2005). Lines running along its side edges should be slightly diverging caudally (Figure 3a). These are commonly described as the dorsal aesthetic lines.

Ideally, the nasal width at nasion should be equal to the palpebral fissure; while at the level of pronasale (width of the nasal base) should be similar to the distance between the inner commissures of the eyes. The width of the base of the nasal osseous pyramid should be 70-80% of the nasal base (Mathes & Hentz, 2006).

The shape of the nasal base and columella should resemble the outline of seagull in flight (gull-wing appearance) (Figure 3b) (Gunter et al., 2007). Its shape is attributable to the columella position, which protrudes slightly below the edges of the nasal alae. The 'trunk of the gull' is the lowest portion of the columella, and the 'wings of the gull' are the outlines of the lower edges of alae. The edges of alae are shaped like a dome, convex in caudal-lateral direction.

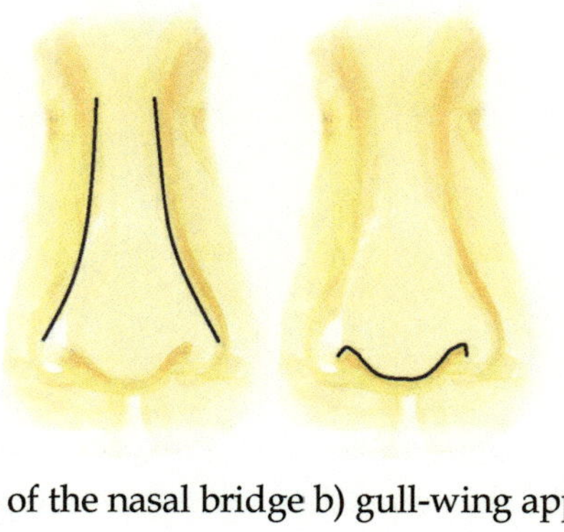

Fig. 3. a) Outline of the edges of the nasal bridge b) gull-wing appearance of the nasal base and columella

In addition, the proportions between the nose and mouth should be considered. The length of the columella should be equal to height of the upper lip (Simons, 1982). Similarly, the upper lip height (distance between subnasale and labiale superius) should be equal to 1/3 of the lower face (1/9 of the whole face, according to the Leonardo da Vinci's canon of beauty) (Trenite, 2005). From the profile, the alar edge should have the shape of the letter 'S', starting at the front of the columella, and ending posteriorly and laterally at the transition between the nasal ala and cheek (Figure 4) (Tardy, 1997).

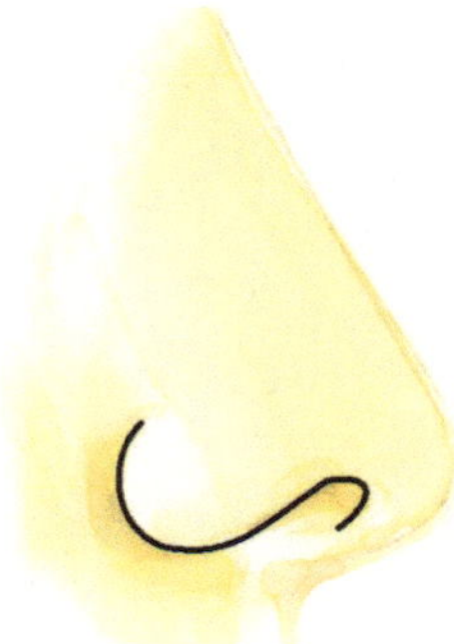

Fig. 4. S-shaped alar edge of the nose

The most attractive nasal profile is straight, as compared to convex or concave. The nasal length and the columella should be proportional, without local irregularities. The nasal profile is well described by the frontonasal angle. The frontonasal angle starts at around eyebrows area and creates a gentle concave arc ending at the bridge of the nose. The top of the frontonasal angle is positioned at level between the free edges of eyelids and supratarsal folds, with eyes opened freely. In women, the nasal profile is straight or slightly concave, in males straight or slightly convex (Tezel & Durmus, 2009).
The nasal tip has two points that define it in the horizontal plane, which are the points on the domes of the nasal alae. Another two points, defining the tip in the profile view, are supratip and columellar breakpoints. Supratip breakpoint is the the stepoff from the the plane of the nasal dorsum on profile view at the cephalic aspect of the nasal tip. Columellar breakpoint forms about 2mm anterior part of the columella (Figure 5 a). All four points that define the nasal tip form two equilateral triangles (Figure 5 b) (Daniel, 2009).

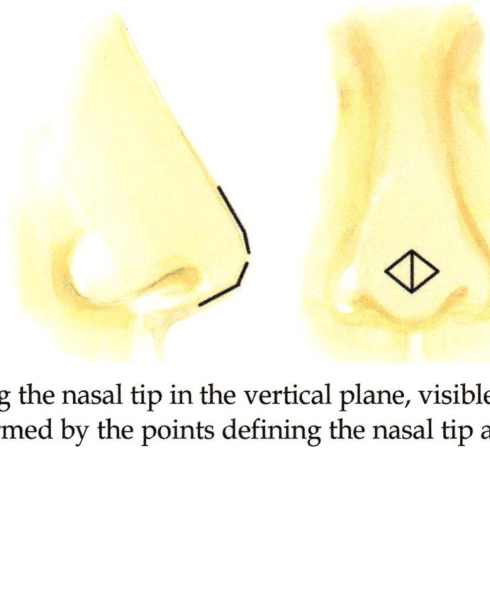

Fig. 5. a) Points defining the nasal tip in the vertical plane, visible from the profile; b) Two equilateral triangles formed by the points defining the nasal tip and the domes of the nasal alae

Projection of the nasal tip is determined by the distance from the junction of the upper lip with alae (subnasale) to the most anterior edge of the nose (pronasale) (Elsahy, 2000). Given the normal projection of the upper lip, 50-60% of this line is located anterior from the most prominent point of the upper lip (Mathes & Hentz, 2006).

Recession of the supratip area is beneficial for women, but does not occur commonly in men. Nasal tip shows more cranial rotation in women (described as supratip break) and therefore is more apparent in females, in contrast to the nasal bridge, which is more prominent in men (Begg & Harkness, 1995).

The worm eye view shows the nasal base. Its external outline in the ideal conditions should create an equilateral triangle (Figure 6). The height of the triangle, measured from the nasal tip (pronasale) to the back of the nose (subnasale) consists of three parts. Its anterior 1/3 passes only through the infratip lobule, whilst the posterior two thirds are located along the columella and nostrils. In another division, its length is divided into two halves at the division of the medial edge of nostrils from the columella. The nostrils have the shape of falling drops, and their widths are similar to the width of the columella. The long axis of the nostrils faces anteriorly and medially about 45 degrees in comparison to the axis of the columella. The width of the columella is narrow in its central part, and widens posteriorly, which reflects the anatomy of the medial crura of alar cartilages. Anteriorly the columella changes into the infratip lobule, whilst posteriorly it connects to the upper lip (Elsahy, 2000).

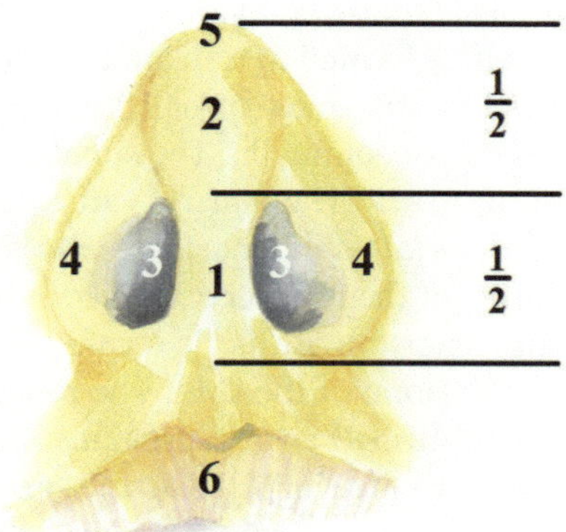

Fig. 6. Base of the nose; 1 - columella, 2 - infratip lobule, 3 - nostrils, 4 - alae, 5 - nasal tip, 6 - upper lip

2.4 Anthropometric measurements of the face and nose

The shape of the cartilaginous-osseous skeleton is relatively well depicted on the skin surface due to the closely fitting skin envelope, especially in patients with thin skin. Therefore, it is possible to designate relatively fixed points of surgical anatomy, which are used for preoperative and intraoperative evaluation. After determining points on the face, anthropometric parameters can be taken, which consist of linear measurements with the resulting indicators, angles and spatial parameters (Szychta et al., 2010).

On the face we suggest determination of 24 anthropometrical points (7 separate for left - L and right - R sides), including points describing the nostrils: anterior (naL, naR), posterior (npL, npR), lateral (nlL, nlR) and medial (nmL, nmR), as well as: subalare (sbalL, sbalR), alare (alL, alR), alar curvature point (acL, acR). Nine single points are also determined: pronasale (prn), infratip lobule (il), subnasale (sn), nasion (n), glabella (gl), labiale superius (ls), rhinion (rh), columellar point (cp), stomion (s) and menton (m) (Figure 7).

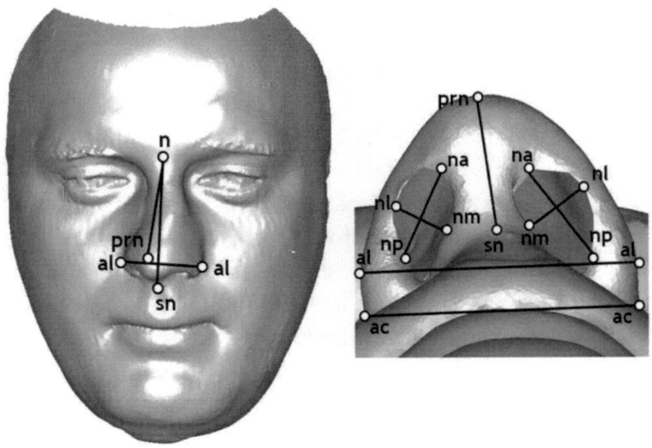

Fig. 7. Anatomical anthropometric points of the face shown on the three-dimensional model of the face; views: a) from the front, b) from the bottom

The nasion (n) is defined in the place of the greatest concavity of the upper pole of the nasal bridge (nasal root). The rhinion (rh) is located at transition of cartilage into osseous pyramid. The pronasale (prn) is described as the most projecting point at the nasal profile. The subnasale (sn) is defined by the base of columella. The subalare (sbal) is located at transition of the ala into the inferior wall of nostril. The alar curvature point (ac) is located in the far lateral basal part of the ala. The alare (al) is the most laterally situated point of the nose. The columellar point (cp) is determined at the intersection of both axes of nostrils, usually being the lowest point of the nasal tip. The stomion (s) is located at the level of the lips fissure, whilst the menton (m) is the lowest point of the chin. The reliability of measurements using the anatomical points has been confirmed in the previous studies. The above mentioned anthropometric points can be used to obtain: 9 linear measurements, 7 indicators of nasal proportions, 7 angles, 2 indicators of spatial asymmetry of the skin surface and the total volume of the operated area.

The linear measurements include: length and width of both nostrils (naR-npR, naL-npL, nlR-nmR and nlL-nmL, respectively), nasal height (n-sn), nasal length (n-prn), nasal width (alL-alR), length of the nasal base (acL-acR) and the nasal prominence (sn-prn). Nasal length (n-prn) should be equal to the distance between stomion and menton (s-m). Nasal height is equal to the length of the upper lip or up to 50% longer. Nasal prominence (sn-prn) is about 2/3 of the nasal length (n-prn). The degree of projection of the nasal tip, determined by the distance sn-prn, should be equal to the upper lip height.

The calculated linear indices are: the index of the nasal base (sn-prn/ac-ac * 100), the index of the prominence to the nasal width (sn-prn/al-al * 100), indicators of the shape of both nostrils (nl-nm/na-np * 100), nasal index (al-al/n-sn * 100) and index of the nasal length (n-prn/n-sn * 100). Asymmetry in the shape of the nostrils is given by [2 * ((nlL-nmL/naL-npL) - (nlR-nmR/naR-npR)) / ((nlL-nmL/naL-npL) + (nlR-nmR/naR-npR)) * 100]. The nasal index is normally 55%-60%.

The analysed angles are: interaxial angle (sbalR-cp-sbalL), angle of deviation between cutaneous septum and midline (cp-sn-median line), angle of deviation between osseous pyramid and midline (rh-n-median line), angle of deviation between osseous and cartilaginous pyramid (n-rh-prn), nasofrontal (gl-n-prn), nasolabial (cp-sn-ls) and nasofacial (n-prn-sn) (Figure 8).

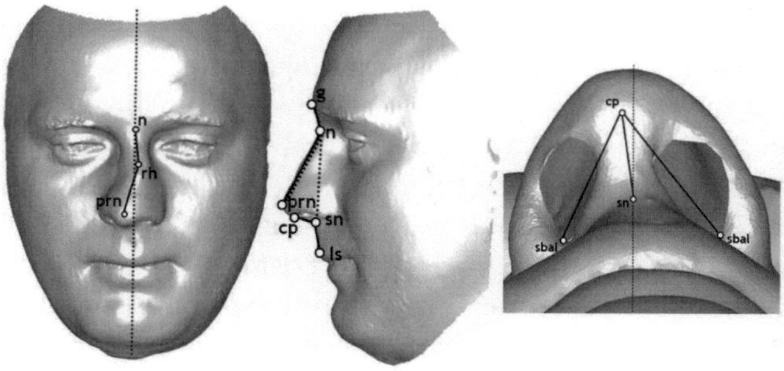

Fig. 8. Angles of the nose, shown on the three-dimensional model of the face; views: a) from the front, b) lateral profile, c) from the bottom

The nasofrontal angle is normally 125-135 degrees. However, the following features of the nasofrontal angle are important for the whole aesthetics of the nose, apart from its value: position of its tip in the frontal and sagittal plane, and its slope. In fact, the nasofrontal angle does not contain a clearly identified vertex, but describes a mild change in the nasal profile. The nasolabial angle in women is 95-105 degrees, while in men it varies from 90 to 95 degrees (Gruber & Peck, 1993). The nasolabial angle directly sets the rotation of the nose. It may be different from the columella-lip angle, e.g. the prominent edge of the caudal nasal septum can cause an illusion of increased cranial rotation of the nose, although the nasolabial angle may remain within normal limits. The nasofacial angle, determining the slope of the nasal bridge of the nose, sets the deviation of the nasal bridge from the facial plane and varies correctly from 34 to 35 degrees (Daniel & Farkas, 1988). An excessively obtuse nasofacial angle indicates excessive projection of the nose, and a very sharp nasofacial angle is often found e.g. in boxers.

Spatial measurements are only possible by using three-dimensional imaging, which has increasing clinical application. Asymmetry of the side surfaces of the nose is described as: [2 * (left side skin surface area - area right) / (area left + area right) * 100], while the asymmetry of cross-sectional areas of the nostrils is equal to [2 * (left cross-section area -area right) / (area left + area right) * 100]. Automated measurement of the total volume of the nose can also be performed (Szychta et al., 2010).

Certainly not all patients will require undergoing the whole abovementioned extensive formal analysis. Such exhaustive measurements are usually important in revision or cosmetic cases with a high degree of precision required. That said, it is important for surgeons to have a working understanding of all of these parameters.

3. The functionality of the nose

3.1 The nasal valve

Internal nasal valve is defined as that area of maximal narrowing that is bounded by the nasal septum, caudal aspect of the upper lateral cartilage, the anterior face of the inferior turvinate and the nasal floor. It is located at a distance of about 1.3 cm posterior to the nostrils (Trenite, 2005). A narrowed nasal valve is the most common cause of reduced patency of the nasal airway, caused by the distortion of the nasal anatomy. Air resistance in the nasal passages may also be caused by incorrect construction of the nasal vestibule or the pathology of the nasal cavity valve.

The external nasal valve, formed by the nasal vestibule caudal to the internal nasal valve, is defined by the alar and lower lateral cartilage tissues, which create the lateral and anterior walls, as well as by the caudal septum and piriform aperture.

Cottle's test is used to detect internal nasal valve pathology (Trenite, 2005). The surgeon places his hand on the patient's cheek near the nasal bridge and then pulls the skin in the lateral direction. In case of valve failure, the patient feels immediate relief on breathing after previous breathing difficulties (positive result). A negative result usually indicates either lack of any pathology in the absence of nasal resistance or a correct nasal valve with pathology of the other area of the nose. A false positive result is found in case of nasal alae collapse. False negative results occur in cases of stenosis or adhesions of the valve or medial displacement of the frontal process of maxilla as a result of mechanical trauma or surgery (Krzeski, 2005).

Another way to evaluate the nasal valve is the introduction of the blunt instrument (e.g. speculum) to the vestibule, moving away the nasal side wall from the septum. Improved function of the nose on inspiration demonstrates pathology of the valve (Krzeski, 2005). Nasal valve collapse is corrected with cartilage grafts. Nasoscopy and cross-sectional imaging have value in illustrating the cause of airway obstruction.

3.2 The mechanism supporting the nose

The cartilaginous-osseous skeleton provides the nasal scaffolding and supports the covering soft tissue (Figure 9). Understanding the mechanisms supporting the nose contributes to an optimal range of surgical manipulation, including the ability to predict correctly the postoperative appearance of the nose after wound healing.

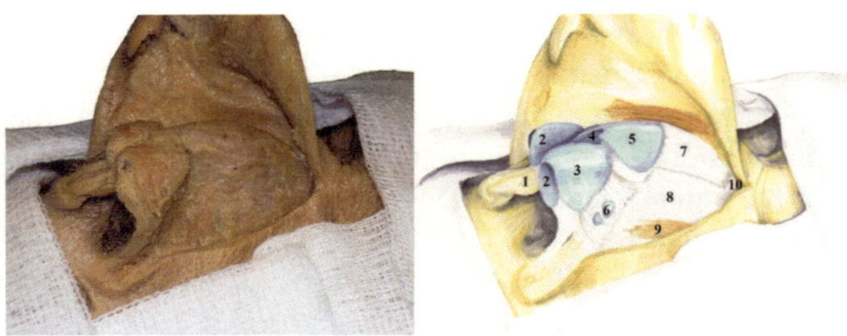

Fig. 9. The cartilaginous-osseous skeleton acting as a support mechanism of the nose: a) cadaveric dissection b) scheme depicting the anatomical details: 1 - skin septum, 2 - medial crus of nasal ala, 3 - lateral crus of nasal ala, 4 - nasal septum, 5 - upper lateral cartilage, 6 - pisiform cartilage, 7 - nasal bone, 8 - frontal process of maxilla, 9 - nasal muscle, 10 - nasal part of frontal bone

There are several mechanisms to support the nose with different significance for individual patients. However, there are three relatively stable mechanisms, which have the greatest impact on the stability of the nasal tip: a) Medial and lateral alar crura (size, shape and structure), b) Ligamentous attachment between the upper lateral nasal cartilages and the alae, and c) Connections between the medial crura of alae and the septum. The less important six elements supporting the nose include: a) ligamentous connection of the alar domes, b) the nasal septum, c) the pisiform cartilages, extending a support function of the lateral crura of alae to the pyriform aperture, d) adhesions of the alae to the covering muscle and skin, e) the nasal spine and f), the membranous septum (Figure 9) (Tardy, 1997). It should be noted that the classic three major support mechanisms are not always the major contributors in all patients. For example, in patients with a tension nose, the nasal septum usurps much of the supporting role of the tip, and may be the single most important support mechanism.

The mechanism for support for the nose can be assessed by checking the 'reversing mechanism'. The nasal tip is squeezed by the thumb and after a rapid withdrawal of the finger the tissue is observed to return to baseline. A slow or incomplete return to the original shape may indicate a weak support apparatus.

Operations, which maintain the structural integrity, result in controlled postoperative outcome. A skeleton of sufficient strength maintains its functional support of the skin, subcutaneous tissue, and SMAS. Moreover, larger noses after subtle correction may be more aesthetically pleasing than small noses after radical reduction. Favourable outcome of nasal correction can be achieved in most cases with conservative reorientation of the anatomical elements.

4. Nasal deformities

4.1 Deviation of the nasal septum

Deviation of the nasal septum should be assessed in the context of the whole nasal skeleton (Figure 10). It often coexists with distortion of the nasal pyramid. The surgeon assesses the visible distortion and examines for fractures using the speculum.

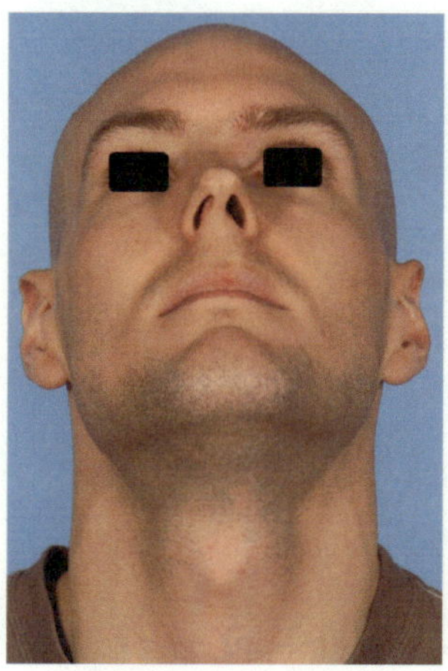

Fig. 10. Twisted nasal septum

4.2 Distortion of the nasal pyramid

Distortion of the nasal pyramid, resulting in impaired function, is a frequent clinical problem, both functionally and aesthetically. In case of deformation of the nasal skeleton, the primary aim is improved breathing. A second aim is correction of nasal aesthetics. A crooked nose is often difficult to repair due to the distorted and scarred skeletal elements and necessitates bilateral surgical manoeuvres to restore symmetry. The importance of the nasal septum in the pathogenesis and the subsequent persistence of crooked nose deformity after surgery should be emphasized. The septum is much like the rudder of a boat. If it is deviated and not corrected, it will steer the nose back to a crooked position even after corrective osteotomies are performed.

Diagnosed type of distortion of nasal pyramid	Distortion of the cartilaginous-osseous skeleton in relation to the median facial line	Shape of the nasal bridge	Position/s of the nasal bridge bend/s
Oblique nose	The cartilaginous and osseous arch veers in the same direction	Straight line	Nasion
Distortion of the cartilaginous pyramid	The osseous pyramid is straight, the cartilaginous pyramid distorted laterally	Singly twisted curve	Rhinion
C-shaped distortion of the nose	The cartilaginous vault is shifted in the opposite direction to the osseous pyramid	Arch	Rhinion and nasion
S-shaped distortion of the nose	The cartilaginous vault shifted in the opposite direction to the osseous pyramid	Double-twisted curve	Nasion, rhinion and area of weakened triangle

Table 1. Division of nasal pyramid deformation, depending on the distortion of the nasal bridge from the midline

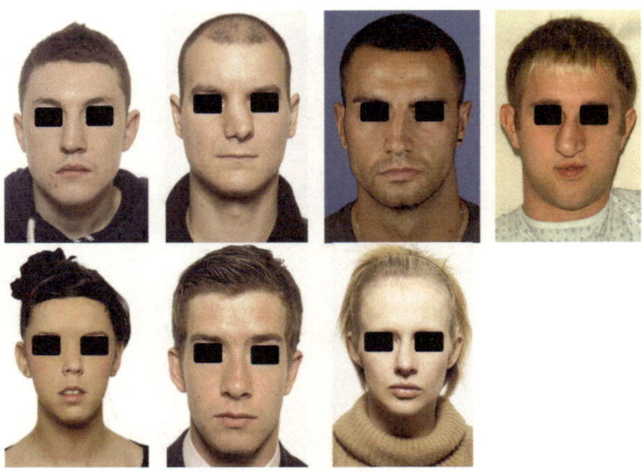

Fig. 11. Division of nasal pyramid deformation, depending on the distortion of the nasal bridge from the midline; a) oblique nose, b) nose with distorted cartilaginous vault, c) 'C'-shaped nose, d) 'S'-shaped nose

Post-traumatic deformity reflects the type and direction of injury. In terms of the extent of cartilaginous and/or osseous damage this may include: a) distortion of the nasal cartilaginous vault by a deviated nasal septum, b) distortion of the entire cartilaginous-osseous skeleton, or c) displacement of the osseous nasal pyramid. Distortion of the external nose, depending on the type of deviation of the nasal bridge from the midline, is described as: a) an oblique nose, b) a hooked nose, c) a saddle nose, or d) and e) 'C' or 'S' shaped nose (Table 1, Figure 11) (Krzeski, 2004). Assessment of the extent of injury helps in planning the appropriate surgical technique. Preoperative evaluation and the subsequent surgical correction should consider separately the three parts of the nose: cranial, middle, caudal.

4.3 The hooked nose

The nasal bridge is built of bone and cartilage. The osseous part is formed by the paired nasal bones, and the cartilaginous is built of lateral nasal cartilages attached to the nasal septum. Their correct proportions define the aesthetics of the nasal bridge. In women this is a straight or slightly concave, whilst in men forms a straight or gently curved line. The nasal hump is an excessive bulge which creates a hooked appearance (Figure 12). The aim of resection of the hump is aesthetic correction that will reconstruct the optimal nasal proportions (Sevin A et al., 2006).

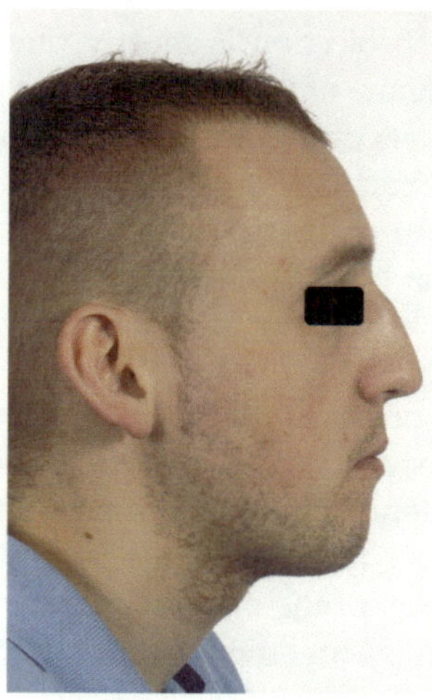

Fig. 12. Hooked nose (nasal hump)

Various anatomical structures may contribute to the nasal hump. These include the osseous pyramid and the cartilaginous vault. However, a genuinely pronounced nose may also give the illusion of a hump. Alleged hump (also called pseudo hump, usually resembling a hump of the osseous pyramid) results from the reduced projection of the upper cartilaginous vault or ptotic tip, giving the impression of excessive convexity of the caudal edge of the nasal bones. The prominent nose includes hypertrophy of the septum cartilage in the sagittal plane and the accompanying hypertrophy of the lateral cartilages of the nose (Krzeski, 2004).

4.4 Saddle nose

The saddle nose is determined by collapse of the nasal bridge, often colloquially described as a 'boxer's nose' or 'puggy nose' (Figure 13).

The saddle nose can be congenital but it is more often acquired. Aetiologies include: iatrogenic cause, certain types of cleft lip and palate, genetic syndromes, congenital syphilis, recurrent cartilaginous inflammation, Wegener's granulomatosis, cocaine use or leprosy.

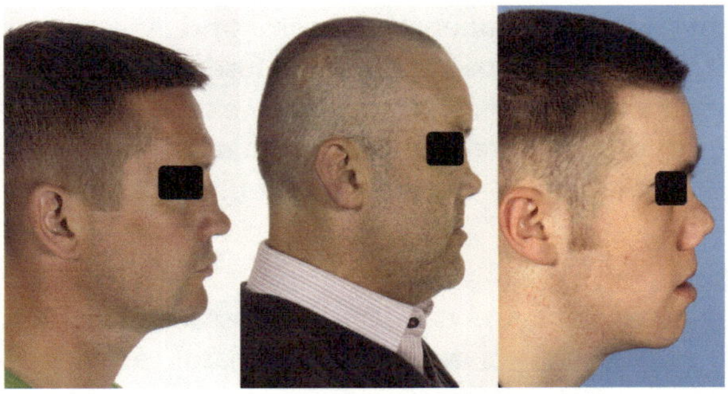

Fig. 13. Saddle nose

A practical method of classification described by Tardy divides severity of the saddle nose deformity into three categories:

a. Minimal - recession of tip supratip area is larger than the ideal 1-2mm, no retraction of the columella, the nose is not widened.
b. Moderate - loss of the nasal projection is mostly due to the damage to nasal septum cartilage. Damage to the cartilage of the nasal septum is a direct cause of weakening of two of the support mechanisms of the nose: the attachment of the medial alar crura to the caudal edge of the septal cartilage and the upper lateral cartilage attachment to the nasal alae. This is the reason for the reduced projection of the nose. The columella is retracted. The pyramid of the nose is too broad and flattened. The nasolabial angle is usually less than 90 degrees. In contrast, the nasal valve angle is often found increased, in rare cases up to 90 degrees.
c. Significant - significant loss of cartilage and loss of projection of the nasal bridge. In cases of a high degree of distortion, the following coexisting distortions are found: a lowered nasal bridge, a shortened columella, loss of support of the nasal tip, shortened nasal length, excessive cranial rotation of the nasal tip, widened nasal tip, alae too prominent and slender, atrophy of the nasal spine and the caudal edge of nasal septum. A decreased nasal tip projection together with a shortened columella is the cause of a disproportionately widened nasal base (Tardy, 1997).

4.5 Distorted nasal tip

The nasal tip is the most prominent area of the nose. Distorted proportions significantly aesthetically influence the facial aesthetics. A larger nose, harmonious with the face is often regarded as more acceptable than the insufficiently prominent one.

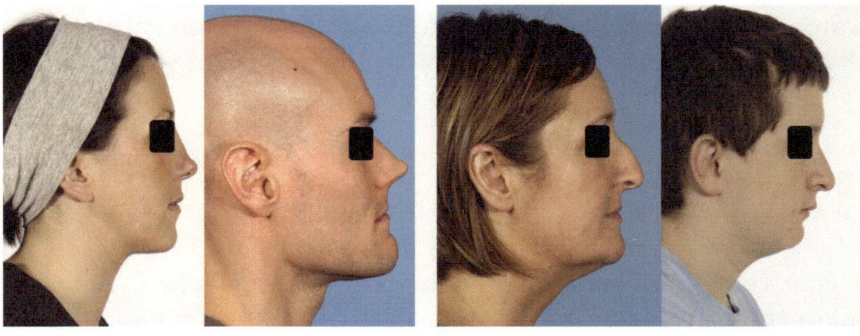

Fig. 14. Rotated nasal tip in women and men; a) snub nose b) droopy nose

In addition to the position, the tip is also determined by caudal or cranial rotation. Excessive cranial rotation, providing a 'snub nose' is acceptable for women and unacceptable in men (Figure 14). On the contrary, 'hanging nose', caused by excessive caudal rotation, is more acceptable in men (Begg & Harkness, 1995). It is often referred to in women as a 'witch nose'.

The supratip area is located between alae and the lateral cartilages. It is filled with adipose tissue. Insufficient volume of this structure can contribute to increased cranial rotation.

5. Consultation of the patient

Rhinoplasty is performed to obtain a functional nose of the correct proportions. Surgeons should acquire the ability to assess the executable range of corrections of the nose, having imposed the pre-established limits. These include anatomical features, such as the characteristics of the covering skin (thickness, elasticity, existing scar tissue), and the cartilaginous-osseous skeleton. In addition, the surgeon should note the areas of the well-proportioned nose, avoiding the changes during the operation (Tardy, 1997).

5.1 Taking a history

On the first visit, the surgeon evaluates the preoperative indication for rhinoplasty, faces the patient's expectations and confronts them with limited operational capability because of the individual anatomical conditions. In the meantime, the surgeon performs the initial analysis of the face and its proportions.

5.1.1 Assessment of patient's motivation

It is essential that the patient himself/herself is convinced of the need for surgery, without pressure from third parties. Recent traumatic experiences in the patient's private or professional life should be regarded as contraindications to surgery. Any signs of body dysmorphic disorder should be also identified. Patient with body dysmorphic disorder focuses usually on one part of the body, most commonly on the nose. His/her preoccupation with an imagined defect in the physical appearance often is expressed as require for surgical correction. The aesthetic outcome of the rhinoplasty is usually not satisfying for these patients with underlying psychiatric disorder (Alavi et al., 2011). The patient qualified for rhinoplasty should be emotionally mature, have realistic expectations about correction and understand his/her contribution to the healing process. With the above conditions of selection, the patients in most cases are happy with a good postoperative result.

By contrast, patients who survived a major injury to the nose are a distinct group of people. For the most patients, they never have considered undergoing surgery without the emergence of posttraumatic deformities to the nose and the related disorder of nasal patency. They want to breathe without difficulty and to have the shape of their nose reconstructed from period before injury. Their motivation is high and usually results in a positive reaction to rhinoplasty (Dziewulski et al., 1995).

The surgeon should be able to identify patients who may pose significant potential problems. These include patients: with unrealistic expectations, hyperaesthetic, obsessive-compulsive, depressive, fickle, hesitant, rude, overly flattering, chummy, sloppy, non-cooperating, 'VIP', overly talkative or haggling over the price of treatment (Tardy, 1997). It should be emphasized that most patients have realistic expectations and understand limited possibilities of correction.

5.1.2 Taking a history – nose

At the beginning of the interview, the surgeon obtains information on conditions that may interfere with nasal function, taking into account: the patency of both nostrils, nasal trauma, seasonal allergies causing nasal obstruction, purulent sinusitis requiring antibiotics, snoring, epistaxis, asthma, headache caused by sinus, bronchitis, history of rhinoplasty or septoplasty, hypertension, tendency to keloids, drugs (aspirin, steroid sprays, decongestants), environmental conditions - work, addictions: cigarettes, alcohol and cocaine (Krzeski, 2004). There is potential of exacerbation of some of these diseases after the surgery. The above mentioned drugs should be discontinued at least one week prior to surgical treatment. Stimulants significantly impair wound healing and can lead to increased incidence of complications. Allergic rhinitis, causing obstruction of the nose, may be due to the hypertrophic inferior nasal turbinates. On this account, the history of headache should not be ignored, as it can exist due to insufficient warming of air inhaled by the inferior nasal turbinates.

Secondly, the surgeon asks questions about patient's concerns in relation to nasal deformations, allowing him/her to answer freely in order to understand the expectations and to assess of executable potential of the requests.

Preliminary analysis of the major complaints gradually shall turn into an assessment of less significant problems. Sometimes patients can not accurately identify problems. Then the surgeon acts as a guide, helping the patient for self-analysis of irregularities by using his experience and artistic sense. Useful descriptors include the words 'harmony' and 'proportion'. To better explain the operative plan to the patient, the surgeon demonstrates certain existing distortions of the individual nose, such as asymmetry, deformities of the nasal tip, distortion of the supratip area, irregularities of the nasal pyramid and nasal septal perforations. It is emphasized that rhinoplasty does not improve the facial symmetry. Sometimes it may become even more apparent after creating a symmetrical nose (Figure 15).

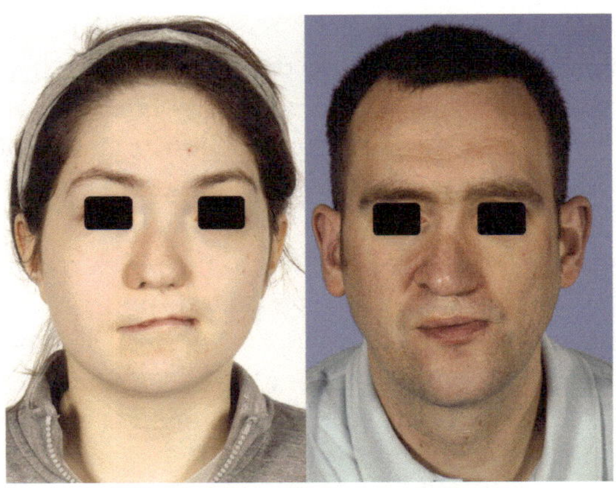

Fig. 15. Asymmetrical faces where rhinoplasty is contraindicated

The first visit should be completed by a thorough understanding between the surgeon and the patient of the aesthetic concerns and opportunities. It is followed by depiction of the operational plan, based on the realistic possibilities of correction of the distorted anatomical components, but also maintaining some of the existing pre-operative characteristics of a desirable nasal shape. In patients without respiratory distress, the surgeon should have in mind the need to maintain the functionality of the nose after surgery.

5.1.3 Preoperative information

Most patients are highly motivated and, after giving the relevant information, do not require a second preoperative interview. Before being asked for the formal consent, they should be informed about possible complications: bleeding, infection, distortion of results from the negative healing, the potential need for reoperation, which may not be possible until 1 year after the first procedure. However, the surgeon should reassure patients that rhinoplasty is usually a relatively safe operation, and that some minor irregularities may disappear in the process of healing.

In the event of the patient deciding to proceed, the surgeon should obtain written consent and photographic documentation. The patient receives a written recommendation concerning the necessary laboratory tests and guidance prior to surgery. Patients often want information about anaesthesia, operative time, length of hospital stay and early postoperative period. They should be informed about the possibility of postoperative pain, swelling of the face, bruising around the eyelids, difficulty in breathing through the nose due to anterior packing and the dressing left for up to seven days. In the case of the planned osteotomy patients should be warned about the need to swap glasses for contact lenses for 6 weeks after surgery.

5.2 The physical examination of the external nose

The surgeon examines the external nose and nasal cavity. At the beginning, an overall evaluation of nasofacial harmony is conducted. Examination of the external nose includes observation and palpation. Firstly, the skin covering the nose is assessed. Then, a systematic analysis of the nose is performed, including the following areas in the caudal direction: the nasofrontal angle, osseous pyramid, the upper lateral cartilage and nasal tip (the supratip area, nasal tip, alae, columella).

5.2.1 Evaluation of nasal skin and subcutaneous tissue

The surgeon can relatively easily modify the nasal cartilage and bone, but the nature of the covering skin must be accepted and included in the technique used for correction. Individual characteristics of each patient's skin have a huge impact on the scope of executable operations and the final result. Nasal skin is resistant to varying degrees to changes in cartilaginous-osseous skeletal, depending on its thickness, texture and elasticity. The elasticity of the skin is reduced in the elderly. The constraints due to the volume of preoperative skin with reduced elasticity must be taken into account during preoperative planning. For example, the skin over a broad nasal base may not contract adequately to cover a small, narrow base of the nose, and the postoperative result rather turns into a distorted wide base of the nose.

The skin is assessed by observation and palpation, checking the extent of the possible surgical correction. Gently lifting the nasal skin allows for an evaluation of its mobility in relation to the nasal skeleton and for the indirect analysis of its elasticity and contractility.

The thickness of the skin is the single most important parameter of the skin. Nasal skin is generally thinner, more mobile, easier shifting in the cranial area, while being relatively devoid of subcutaneous tissue and sebaceous glands. The caudal part of the nose contains a thicker skin more strongly attached to the substrate, with a higher content of the sebaceous glands. Skin is thickest in the following areas: the nasal root (nasion), supratip area, whiles the thinnest at the rhinion (Krzeski, 2005). This should be taken into account when considering nasal reduction. Nasal tip contains additional subcutaneous tissue.

The best skin for the perfect result of rhinoplasty is of moderate thickness. It consists of the epidermis that includes minimum number of sebaceous glands and pores. Sufficient quantity of fibrous tissue and fat protects the skin from underlying skeletal structures, while hiding minor irregularities in the nasal cartilages. It adheres well to the bed after the surgery, so that changes made to the skeleton translate into the desired changes in the appearance of soft tissue.

In patients with thin, delicate skin, less postoperative swelling and fast wound healing are observed (Figure 16 a). However, it does not disguise small irregularities in the skeleton, making the shape of the nose edgy and unnatural. In most patients, the skin is medium thick or thin, so the surgeon should make every effort to save the subcutaneous tissue during operation (Tardy, 1997).

Thicker nasal skin is un-aesthetic (Figure 16 b). For those with thicker skin, a higher postoperative swelling is observed, together with slower healing and more pronounced contraction. The creation of scar tissue under the skin is more pronounced, especially for a nasal reduction. This leads to a parrot nose (pollybeak), a shapeless nose. It is difficult to obtain the accentuated definition of the nose in patients with thick nasal skin. After the operation is adheres poorly to the nasal skeleton. Care should also be taken not to resect excessively the cartilaginous skeleton due to the danger of weakening the support of the nose (Mathes & Hentz, 2006).

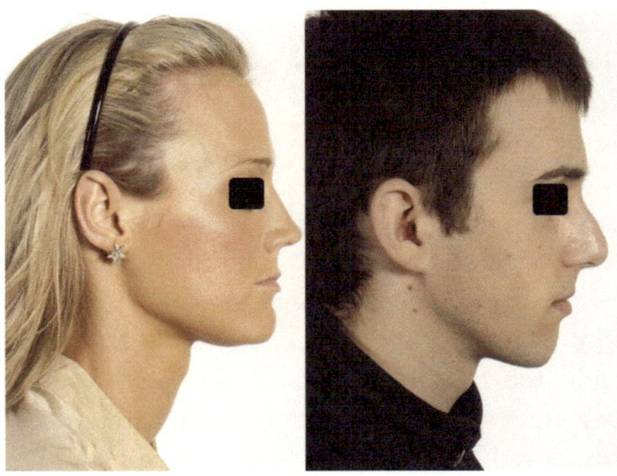

Fig. 16. Noses with a) thin, b) thick nasal skin

5.2.2 Examination of the cartilaginous-osseous nasal skeleton

Ability to assess the external shape of the nose during the physical examination is largely dependent on knowledge of the topographical points of the face and nose, as well as classic proportions described by Leonardo da Vinci. However, often the practical usefulness of these aesthetic purposes is limited by the anatomy of skeleton and the surrounding skin.

The examination is performed in an orderly manner, in caudal direction (Elsahy, 2000). The surgeon evaluates the location and slope of the frontonasal and nasolabial angles. Frontonasal angle can be improperly shifted cranially or caudally, so the nose is elongated or abnormally short. Too mild frontonasal angle is an indication for resection of bone or longitudinal muscle. If too sharp, it forms a clearly visible vertex of the frontonasal angle, which is an indication for the cartilage graft (Figure 17).

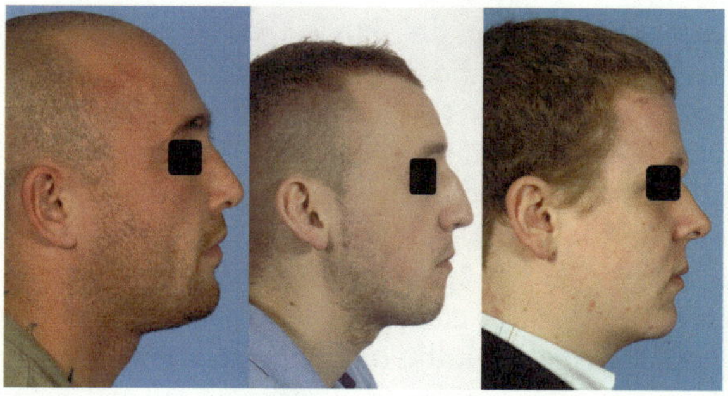

Fig. 17. Frontonasal angle; a) obtuse, b) normal, c) acute

Nasal bones are examined for symmetry, the occurrence of irregularities and their length. It is important to determine the ratio between the width of the base of the nose and the length of the bridge (Elsahy, 2000). Simultaneously, visual illusion must be taken into account on the inverse relation between the projection of the nasal bridge and the size of the nasal base (Figure 18). The aim is to select the optimum reduction of osseous pyramid or augmentation of the area.

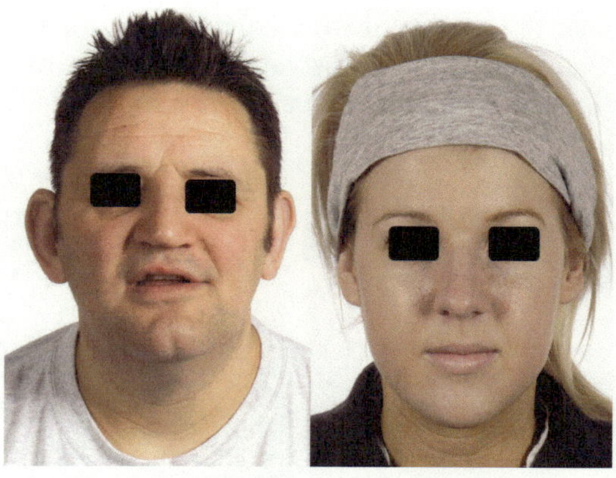

Fig. 18. Two noses with the similar length and a) wider b) narrower nasal base - visual illusion of the shorter nose in the picture on the left because of the wider nasal base

The surgeon assesses the lateral cartilages in terms of their symmetry and strength. Lateral nasal cartilages are compared with nasal bones and nasal septum cartilage in order to assess their supportive function. For shorter nasal bone, the weaker support of the nasal valve is experienced. In these cases, only conserving hump removal can be performed in order to avoid the collapse of the lateral cartilages (Gunter et al., 2007).

Assessment of stiffness and support to the lower third of the nose is of crucial importance in the multivariate analysis of the nose. In order to assess valve pathology, the patient is asked to breathe intensively. The surgeon observes collapsing or asymmetry in the nasal side walls, the distortion of the columella, protrusion of the caudal part of nasal septum or collapse of the alae. Reliable screening test (evaluation of 'reversing mechanism') to denote the support of mobile bottom third of the nose consists of strong pressing of the nasal tip to the upper lip using your finger tip, and subsequent sudden release. Then the ability of the nasal tip return to baseline is observed (Krzeski, 2005).

Nasal base is a more complex structure compared to the simple structure of the osseous and upper cartilaginous vaults. In addition, the skin in the caudal pole of the nose is thicker and thus less adapted to surgical manipulation.

Supratip area is evaluated in terms of its position (height, width and recession) and symmetry. In normal conditions it should be flat.

The nasal tip is examined in terms of its projection, rotation, symmetry and position of defining points. Identification of poorly defined tip, a low point of greatest projection tip, convex supratip area, infratip lobule lying above the point of greatest projection helps in planning a thorough correction of this complex anatomical structure.

Nasal alae are examined in terms of width, retraction, and place of connection to columella. The abnormal curvature or asymmetry can be observed. Visual inspections on a peaceful and forceful breathing allow to depict collapse, flaccidity of the cartilage or narrowing of the nasal valve. Palpation determines their size, mobility, shape and strength. The increased distance between the domes of the alae is an indication for correcting the forked nasal tip (Elsahy, 2000).

Infratip lobule is assessed in terms of shape, harmony with the surrounding structures, width, thickness and the ratio of the nasal length and the nasal base width.

Nostrils are assessed in terms of shape and symmetry (Figure 19). At the same time, shape of columella is observed. Examination of columellar width and length allows to assess its supportive function. In case of too short medial crura of alae, there is a need of longitudinal, narrow cartilage graft. Correction of excessive tip projection may include reducing the width and length of too long or widening medial crura of nasal alae (Gunter et al., 2007).

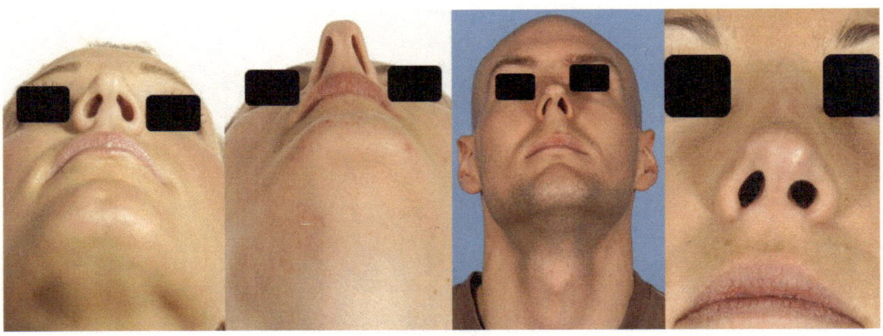

Fig. 19. Shape of nostrils: a) symmetrical teardrop-shaped, b) symmetrical narrow, c) asymmetrical in width, d) asymmetrical in length

The nasolabial angle is examined by observation. Excessively acute angle (less than 80 degrees) indicates a drooping nasal tip - on the assumption that there is no evidence of 'hanging columella' (Figure 20). Excessively acute or retracted nasolabial angle is an indication for tip reduction or transplantation thickening grafts (called plumping grafts) at intersection of columella and the upper lip (subnasale). Excessively obtuse angle is more challenging to repair and requires usually cartilage or bone graft (Krzeski, 2005).

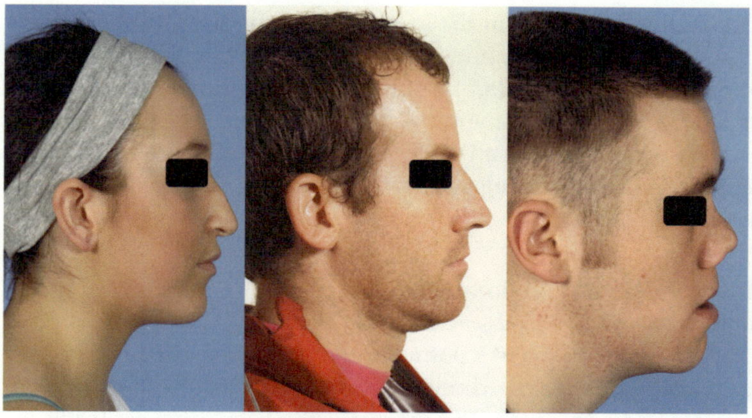

Fig. 20. Nasolabial angle; a) excessively acute, b) normal, c) excessively obtuse

Septal cartilage is examined from the outside in terms of its relation to columella. Palpation is performed with thumb and index finger, allowing to check twisted caudal edge of nasal septum, hypertrophic cartilage septum, caudal distortion of the medial alar crura and columella or structural abnormalities of the anterior nasal spine (Figure 21).

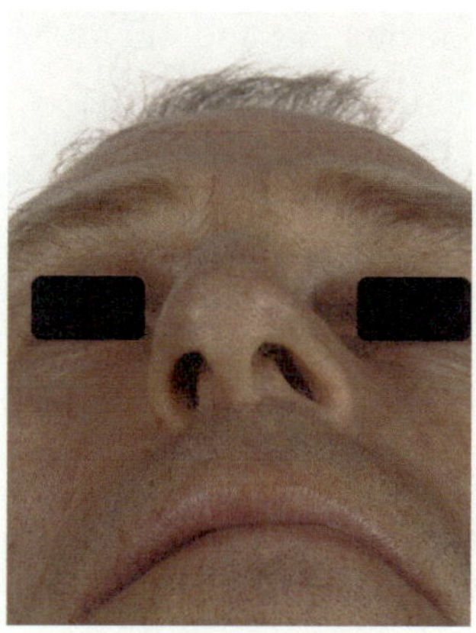

Fig. 21. Distortion of the nasal septum from the midline

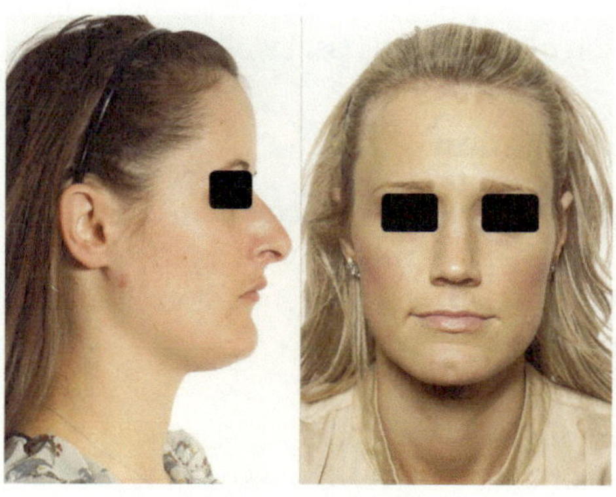

Fig. 22. a) Hanging columella, b) recessed columella

Excessively protruding columella in the lower pole of the nose, or too big alae, resulting in excessive outline of 'gull in flight', are called 'hanging columella' (Figure 22). In contrast, a flat line is called recessed columella. An important point in nasal analysis is differentiating alar retraction from a hanging columella.

The infratip lobule should be localized below the top of the alar domes. Uncommonly observed 'hanging infratip lobule' occurs when infratip lobule has a too low position relative to the junction of alae.

5.3 Examination of the internal nose

Intranasal examination allows to assess the functionality of the nose. It is performed using a speculum, after applying vascular contractile factor in the aerosol (oxymetazoline). The following structures can be assessed: mucosa, nasal turbinates, nasal septum, nasal valve, valve of nasal cavity and nasal ala. The review of the nasal duct confirms nasal patency or indicates the anatomical abnormalities (Tebbetts, 2008).

Assessment of the appearance of mucosa is in consideration of the appearance, atrophic changes, oedema, presence of polyps and anatomical abnormalities in the lateral wall of the nasal cavity.

Nasal turbinates are assessed visually in terms of their size, shape and appearance. Their hypertrophy is common in people with allergies. Because of their functions, the conserving resection should be carried out and only when absolutely necessary (Krzeski, 2004).

Septum is examined to assess its size, shape, coverage of the mucosa, perforation or adhesions. Curvature of the nasal septum posterior from the nasal valve can be detected. Excessive size of septum is noted for its potential use as a graft. Identification of high distortion of the septum (anterior edge) is important to avoid formation of high curvature of the septum after removal of the nasal hump. It is important to detect the curved horizontal cribriform plate because it can cause impaired nasal patency after the lateral osteotomy (Mathes & Hentz, 2006).

Nasal valve can be easily visualized due to its relatively superficial location. Angle of the valve is formed by the nasal septum and lateral nasal cartilage, amounting normally from 10 to 15 degrees (Trenite, 2005). In order to evaluate the nasal valve, the patient's head is tilted back and the surgeon uses a point light source to observe the presence of a narrow valve, or its collapse on inhalation.

Alae are examined to detect the protrusion of their lateral crura to the vestibule and to assess their support function of the lateral nasal wall.

6. Photographic documentation

Pre- and postoperative photographic documentation is a valuable addition to the daily practice of surgeon involved in the rhinoplasty for the following purposes: diagnostic, teaching, self-criticism, as well as medico-legal. Surgeon should obtain written consent from the patient for the photographs to be taken.

6.1 Two-dimensional photographs

Routine photographic documentation on a preoperative visit involves an additional 2 minutes, and provides invaluable information on the nasal shape.

Quality images are obtained using the 105 mm portrait lens (Mathes & Hentz, 2006). Patient should be placed approximately 150 cm from the photographer. Proper lighting provides a set of two lamps directed at an angle of 45 degrees to the camera and the patient. The greatest depth of focus will be provided by optics lens with aperture F-11 to F-22. The background colour should be pale pastel in order to avoid reflection or absorption of an excessive light rays, as well as to be a good complement to the colour of the skin (Tardy, 1997).

Face of the patient should be placed along the Frankfort line. From the front, head and neck should be included. From the side profile, ear and nose should be taken into account. In order to standardize the oblique profile, the lateral border of the face should be adjusted with the tip of the nose. From the bottom, tip of the nose should be positioned between the eyebrows. The patient is placed no closer than 50 cm from the background in order to avoid the shadows.

Normally, six photographs are carried out in the following projections: front (lens at eye level), lateral (left and right profile - invisible opposite eyebrow), oblique (left and right) and the base of the nose (Figure 23).

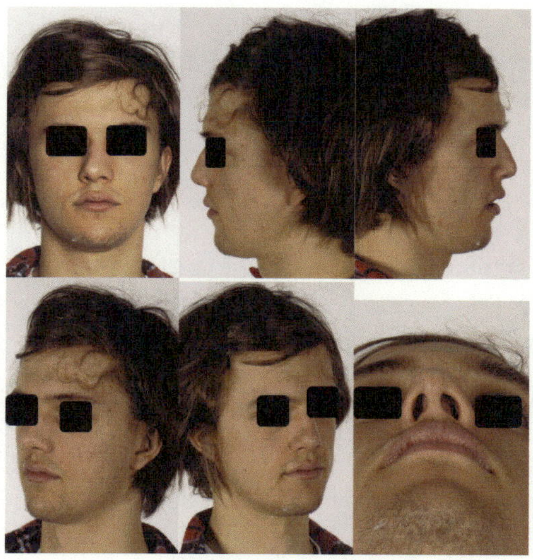

Fig. 23. Routine photographic documentation of the patient prior to rhinoplasty

6.2 Three-dimensional imaging

Three-dimensional imaging method allows to determine the shape of a three-dimensional object (e.g. face). Scanning requires set of devices, which transform the image from analog to digital form and include: an optical system, digital communication network and computer with the calculation program. Image captured by an optical system is subjected to computer analysis in the process of digitization. Body surface area is written in the form of points with coordinates in three dimensions. Points are combined with one another to form triangles on poligonisation. The collection of all triangles in a three-dimensional model forms the surface of analysed part of the body, which contains information concerning its actual size (Figure 24). 3D scanner should be configured to allow an accurate assessment of the linear measurements, proportion, area and volume.

With three-dimensional imaging all currently designated line parameters can be achieved in a repeatable and precise way, as well as additional spatial data describing the shape of the nose, which could be useful for preoperative planning. The postoperative data allow for accurate long-term follow-up. Three-dimensional imaging can also provide invaluable assistance to the surgeon through the preoperative calculation of the needed degree of resection of the nasal cartilages during surgery. Confirmation of usefulness of this method of preoperative planning, however, requires further study.

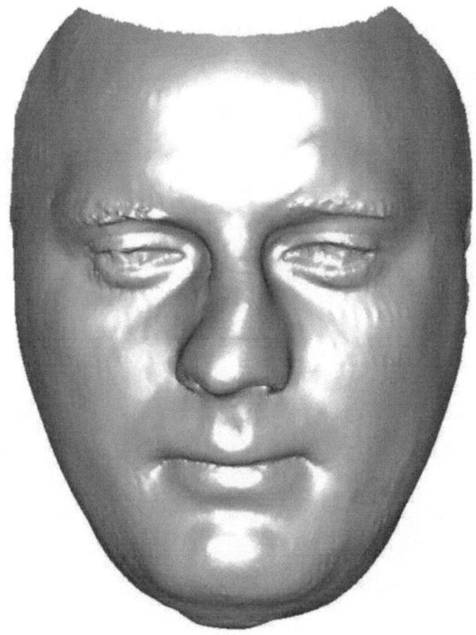

Fig. 24. Three-dimensional model of the face

7. Additional studies

Labolatory tests should be performed two weeks prior to rhinoplasty, these may include: blood group, full blood count, ESR, urea + electrolytes, coagulation tests (INR, APTT), HBV antigen, HCV antibodies.
The following tests may be additionally recommended: WR, total protein, urinalysis, chest X-ray and ECG.

8. Conclusions

Proper selection of patients together with detailed preoperative planning, based on accurate knowledge of the nasal anatomy, is essential to achieve good result of rhinoplasty. The relatively fixed points of the nasal surgical anatomy, designated using our protocol of anthropometrical assessment with 3D imaging, can be used for accurate preoperative and intraoperative evaluation. However, ideal proportions of the nose to the whole face act only as guidelines in individualized planning of the surgery.

9. References

Alavi, M.; Kalafi, Y.; Dehbozorgi, G.R. & Javadpour, A. (2011). Body dysmorphic disorder and other psychiatric morbidity in aesthetic rhinoplasty candidates. Journal of

Plastic, Reconstructive and Aeshtetic Surgery, Vol.64, No.6, (June 2011), pp.738-41, ISSN 1748-6815

Begg, R.J. & Harkness, M. (1995). A lateral cephalometric analysis of the adult nose. Journal of Oral and Maxillofacial Surgery, Vol.53, No.11, (November 1995), pp.1268-1274, ISSN 0278-2391

Daniel, R.K. & Farkas, L.G. (1988). Rhinoplasty: image and reality. Clinics in Plastic Surgery, Vol.15, No.1, (January 1988), pp.1-10, ISSN 0094-1298

Daniel, R.K. (2009). Tip Refinement Grafts: The Designer Tip. Aesthetic Surgery Journal, Vol.29, No.6, (November - December 2009), pp.528-537, ISSN 1084-0761

Dziewulski, P.; Dujon, D.; Spyriounis, P.; Griffiths, R.W. & Shaw J.D. (1995). A retrospective analysis of the results of 218 consecutive rhinoplasties. British Journal of Plastic Surgery, Vol.48, No.7, (October 1995), pp.451-454, ISSN 0007-1226

Elsahy, N. (Ed.). (2000). Plastic and Reconstructive Surgery of the Nose, 1st edn., W.B. Saunders Co., ISBN: 0-7216-7722-3, Philadelphia, USA

Gruber, R.P. & Peck, G.C. (Eds.). (1993). Rhinoplasty: State of the Art, 1st edn., Mosby, ISBN-13 978-0801662775, St. Louis, USA

Gunter, J.P.; Rohrich, R.J. & Adams, W.P. (Eds.). (2007). Dallas Rhinoplasty - Nasal Surgery by the Masters, 2nd edn., Quality Medical Publishing Inc., ISBN-13 978-1-57626-223-8, St. Louis, USA

Krzeski, A. (Ed.). (2004). [Podstawy chirurgii nosa], In Polish. 1st edn., Via Medica, ISBN 83-89861-10-0, Gdansk, Poland

Krzeski, A. (Ed.). (2005). [Wyklady z chirurgii nosa]. In Polish. 1st ed., Via Medica, ISBN 83-89861-29-1, Gdansk, Poland

Mathes, S.J. & Hentz, V.R. (Eds.). (2006). Plastic Surgery. Volume II - The Head and Neck, Part 1, 2nd edn., Saunders Elsevier Inc., ISBN-13 978-0-7216-8811-4, Philadelphia, USA

Perrett, D.I.; May, K.A. & Yoshikawa, S. (1994). Facial shape and judgements of female attractiveness. Nature, Vol.368, No.6468, (March 1994), pp:239-242

Powell, N. & Humphreys, B. (Eds.). (1984). Proportions of the aesthetic face, 1st edn., Thieme-Stratton, ISBN 0865771170, New York, USA

Rahman, M.; Jefferson, N.; Stewart, D.A.; Oliver, R.; Walsh, W.R. & Gianoutsos, M.P. (2010). The histology of facial aesthetic subunits: Implications for common nasal reconstructive procedures. Journal of Plastic, Reconstructive and Aesthetic Surgery, Vol.63, No.5, (May 2010), pp.753-756, ISSN 1748-6815

Sevin, A.; Sevin, K.; Erdogan, B.; Adanali, G. & Deren, O. (2006). A Useful Method for Planning Hump Resection of Deviated Nose. Aesthetic Plastic Surgery, Vol.30, No.4, (August 2006), pp.433-436, ISSN 0364-216X

Simons, R.L. (1982). Nasal tip projection, ptosis, and supratip thickening. ENT - Ear, Nose, & Throat Journal, Vol.61, No.8, (August 1982), pp.452-455, ISSN 0145-5613

Szychta, P.; Rykala, J. & Kruk-Jeromin, J. (2010). Assessment of 3D scanner usefulness in aesthetic evaluation of posttraumatic rhinoplasty. The 33rd European Academy of Facial Plastic Surgery Meeting, (September 2010), Belek, Turkey

Talakoub, L. & Wesley, N.O. (2009). Differences in Perceptions of Beauty and Cosmetic Procedures Performed in Ethnic Patients. Seminars in Cutaneous Medicine and Surgery, Vol.28, No.2, (June 2009), pp.115-129, ISSN 1085-5629

Tardy, M.E. (Ed.). (1997). Rhinoplasty - The Art and the Science, 1st edn., W.B. Saunders Co., ISBN 0-7216-8755-5, Philadelphia, USA
Tebbetts, J.B. (Ed.). (2008). Primary Rhinoplasty - Redefining the Logic and Techniques, 2nd edn., Mosby Elsevier Inc., ISBN 978-0-323-04111-9, Philadelphia, USA
Tezel, E. & Durmus, F.N. (2009). A new instrument for achieving a natural nasofrontal angle. Journal of Plastic, Reconstructive & Aesthetic Surgery, Vol.62, No.12, (December 2009), pp.e617-e619, ISSN 1748-6815
Trenite, G.J.N. (Ed.). (2005). Rhinoplasty: a practical guide to functional and aesthetic surgery, 3rd edn., Kugler Publication, ISBN 90-6299-208-0, Hague, Netherlands

Part 2

Innovations in Delivery Approach

4

Modified Delivery Approach – A New Perspective

Rui Xavier
Hospital da Arrábida, Porto
Portugal

1. Introduction

Every rhinoplasty begins with the analysis of the patient. For this analysis it is very important to carefully assess not only the nose, but also the facial features and the morphological characteristics of the patient´s body. After this evaluation a list of the surgical techniques necessary to achieve the desired nose is drawn and, according to this surgical planning, the surgical approach is selected.

The surgical approach should provide adequate exposure of the nasal structures that are to be addressed by surgery, and should allow the various surgical techniques to be executed without difficulty and without jeopardizing the nasal structures. For providing adequate exposure, however, every approach has to divide or to elevate nasal cartilaginous and soft tissues structures, and this may interfere, to a certain degree, with the natural mechanisms of tip support and strength. Several nasal structures are unanimously recognised as contributing to the tip support. The factors influencing this support are usually classified as the *major* and the *minor* tip support mechanisms. The *major* tip support mechanisms are: the size, shape, thickness and resilience of the alar cartilages; the upper lateral cartilages attachment to the cephalic margin of the alar cartilages; the attachment of the medial crura footplates to the caudal septum. The *minor* tip support mechanisms are: the ligamentous sling spanning the domes of the alar cartilages; the membranous septum; the cartilaginous septal dorsum; the nasal spine; the sesamoid complex extending the support of the lateral crura to the piriform aperture; the attachment of the alar cartilages to the overlying skin and musculature. (3,4).

Recent studies have underscored the role of the upper lateral cartilages attachment to the cephalic margin of the alar cartilages to maintain a strong tip support (5,6). It has been demonstrated that this attachment is made of fibrous tissue consisting of dense collagen fibers, all orientated in a single direction, thus fulfilling the criteria of a true ligament (5).

Another study demonstrated that the most efficient way to release the tip as to be freely moved is severing these fibrous attachments between the upper lateral and the alar cartilages (6), thus highlighting the role of this ligament to the tip support. Every effort should be made, therefore, to preserve these collagen fibres during rhinoplasty, in order not to weaken the support of the nasal tip. This should be kept in mind while performing rhinoplasty, as well as while choosing the approach for surgery.

The three *standard* approaches for rhinoplasty are the non-delivery approach, the delivery approach and the open approach (7).
The non-delivery or cartilage-splitting approach is very suitable to achieve minor modifications of the nasal tip, such as a moderate increase in tip rotation or an improvement in tip definition (3,8,9) and also provides good access to the upper two thirds of the nose, particularly when reduction techniques to the dorsum are being planned. This approach involves only one incision, a transcartilaginous incision.
The non-delivery approach is particularly suitable for patients with reasonable tip symmetry, normal domal angles and normal or almost normal interdomal distance (3). The great advantage of this approach is its simplicity and easiness to perform, with good and predictable results (8), as it causes almost no interference to the natural mechanisms of tip support (7,10).
The delivery approach is an elegant approach that allows more delicate tip work than the non-delivery approach. Two incisions are usually made for this approach: an intercartilaginous incision and a marginal incision.
This intercartilaginous incision may cause scarring at the valve area, if not made slightly caudally to the caudal border of the upper lateral cartilages (9). It may also promote weakening of one of the *major* support mechanisms of the nasal tip, the upper lateral cartilage attachment to the cephalic margin of the alar cartilage (10,11).
Nevertheless, besides providing access to the upper two thirds of the nose, the delivery approach is often used to correct bifidity or asymmetry of the tip, to achieve extra tip rotation or to change tip projection (7,9). With the delivery approach, precise excision of cartilage is possible, as well as it is possible to introduce and fixate cartilaginous grafts. It is also possible to interrupt the continuity of the alar cartilages in order to change nasal tip projection and rotation, or to enhance tip projection with a lateral crura steal (9). The delivery approach allows an excellent exposition of the alar cartilages that may, thus, be remodelled as necessary. This approach is particularly useful in patients with a non triangular tip (on basal view), with wide domal angles and large interdomal distance (3,8).
The open approach uses a marginal incision and an external (columelar) incision. The great advantage of this approach is the superb visual control of every structure of the nasal framework that it allows (7,12,13). Another advantage of the open approach is affording an enhanced surgical exposure, facilitating nasal sculpturing by suturing or by the introduction and fixation of different kind of grafts. Any modification of the cartilages can be performed and the result may be easily assessed. The open approach allows maximal exposure of the tip, improving diagnosis and facilitating correction of gross deformities (11,14,15).
The extra time necessary for the approach and for carefully closing the incisions cannot be considered a drawback of the open approach, and the interference that the open approach causes to the mechanisms of tip support (3,10,13), although relevant, may be overcome by using surgical techniques that reinforce this support at some stage of the procedure (10).
The open approach, however, does leave an extensive submucous wound area, leading to a prolonged edema and to longer healing time (3); there may be sensory disturbances at the tip area and there will be an external scar, which may be of concern for some patients and that, eventually, may not be completely undistinguishable.

Due to its maximal surgical exposure, improved diagnosis and facilitated correction of deformities, the open approach is particularly useful for patients with marked asymmetry of the tip, patients undergoing major reconstruction of the tip or of the upper two thirds of the nose and patients whose complete diagnosis is still unclear after a careful preoperative analysis of the nose (3,9).

The non-delivery approach, the delivery approach and the open approach are the three standard approaches for rhinoplasty. Some surgeons always perform rhinoplasty by using an open approach, others always use an endonasal approach; we believe that every facial plastic surgeon should be familiar with all approaches, as the choice of the approach should not be dictated by the preferences of the surgeon but, mainly, by the nasal deformities of the patient and by the surgical techniques that have been planned in order to achieve an improvement in nasal functioning and aesthetics.

The simplest approach that allows the planned surgical techniques to be performed without difficulty should be selected, to cause the least disturbance to the tip support (3,7,13). The surgeon must always weigh the surgical trauma caused by the approach against the surgical exposure afforded by the approach. In other words, the approach should be as invasive as necessary, but, at the same time, as non invasive as possible.

A frequent goal of rhinoplasty is achieving an improvement in tip definition; for this purpose it is often advisable to resect the cephalic margin of the lateral crura of the alar cartilages, sometimes combining this procedure with other techniques, such as single dome or double dome sutures, or scoring or morselization of the cartilages. The delivery approach is very appropriate to accomplish these manoeuvres, and is widely used (3,9).

If the patient has long alar cartilages (in the cranial-caudal direction), it is particularly important to resect a cephalic piece of the lateral crura to improve tip definition. In this kind of cartilages, however, it may be difficult to deliver the alar cartilages without twisting or tearing the most lateral part of the lateral crura and the intermediate crura or even the dome area. The dome segment is usually the thinnest and most delicate portion of the entire alar cartilage (16) and any weakening of this portion may endanger the resilience of the cartilage, which could compromise the support of the nasal tip. When planning surgery, the open approach may be chosen to overcome this; however, a modified delivery approach may also be used, turning the exposure of the tip cartilages easier and safer, and avoiding using an intercartilaginous incision, which could interfere with the tip support.

2. Surgical technique

For the modified delivery approach a transcartilaginous incision is first used in each side of the nose. The position of this incision must take into account that the exact amount of cartilage to be resected may be difficult to assess at this stage, so care must be taken to leave an appropriated sized cartilage caudal to the incision (figure 1). The cephalic piece of the alar cartilage is dissected free in the vestibular and in the non-vestibular sides and resected (figure 2). This procedure is repeated in the opposite side of the nose.

Then a marginal incision is made (figure 3), and the remaining alar cartilage is dissected in the non-vestibular side and easily delivered (figure 4). After the same procedure is

performed in the opposite side, both alar cartilages are delivered. At this stage of the procedure the size of the remaining alar cartilages is assessed; if necessary, further cephalic resection is done in order to achieve perfect symmetry or to achieve the desired size of the alar cartilages (figure 5).
The rhinoplasty may then proceed with other surgical techniques to the alar cartilages, which may be grafted, sutured or modified as considered necessary to achieve a good functional and aesthetic result (figure 6). After addressing the upper two thirds of the nose, at the end of surgery both the transcartilaginous and marginal incisions are closed with an absorbable suture material.

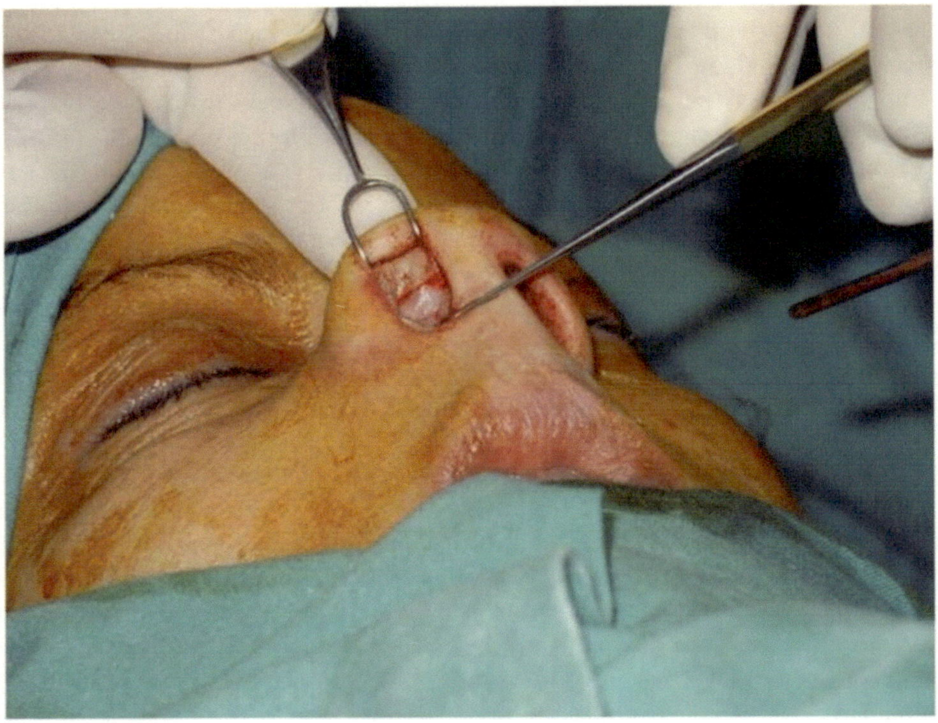

Fig. 1. A transcartilaginous incision is first used, taking care to leave an appropriated sized cartilage caudal to the incision

3. Comments

A large proportion of patients seeking rhinoplasty will benefit from surgery of the nasal tip. This may involve major reconstruction for correction of gross asymmetry or deformity of the tip cartilages, usually achieved by using an open approach. For most patients, however, the nose will benefit from performing slight modifications in tip rotation or projection, from correcting a bifid or boxy tip or from improving tip definition. These modifications can be achieved by using an endonasal approach, usually a delivery approach.
Though very appropriate for performing these surgical manoeuvres, the delivery approach has been criticized by some surgeons, and one of the reasons for this criticism is the intercartilaginous incision usually used for this approach.

If not placed slightly caudal to the caudal border of the upper lateral cartilages, the intercartilaginous incision may lead to scarring of the valve area (9), which could compromise the breathing capacity of the nasal cavity due to narrowing of the internal nasal valve.

We have been using this modified delivery approach for several years without any complications. Several clinical cases of patients operated on by using this approach have previously been reported (1,2).

Another reason for criticizing the intercartilaginous incision is the damage produced by this incision on the collagen fibers situated between the upper lateral cartilages and the cephalic border of the alar cartilages. The importance of the attachment between these cartilages has been well recognized for a long time and considered a *major* tip support mechanism. Recently, this attachment has been described as a true ligament, due to the fact that it is made of dense collagen fibers organised in a single direction (5).

The advantage of this modified approach over the traditional delivery approach is avoiding the intercartilaginous incisions. The dense collagen tissue between the upper lateral and the alar cartilages will not be severed by using a transcartilaginous incision, thus preventing weakening of the tip support. It has been shown that dividing this fibrous tissue has much more effect on releasing tip structures than dividing any other soft tissue important to the tip support mechanisms (6), emphasising the importance of keeping this tissue to maintain a strong tip support.

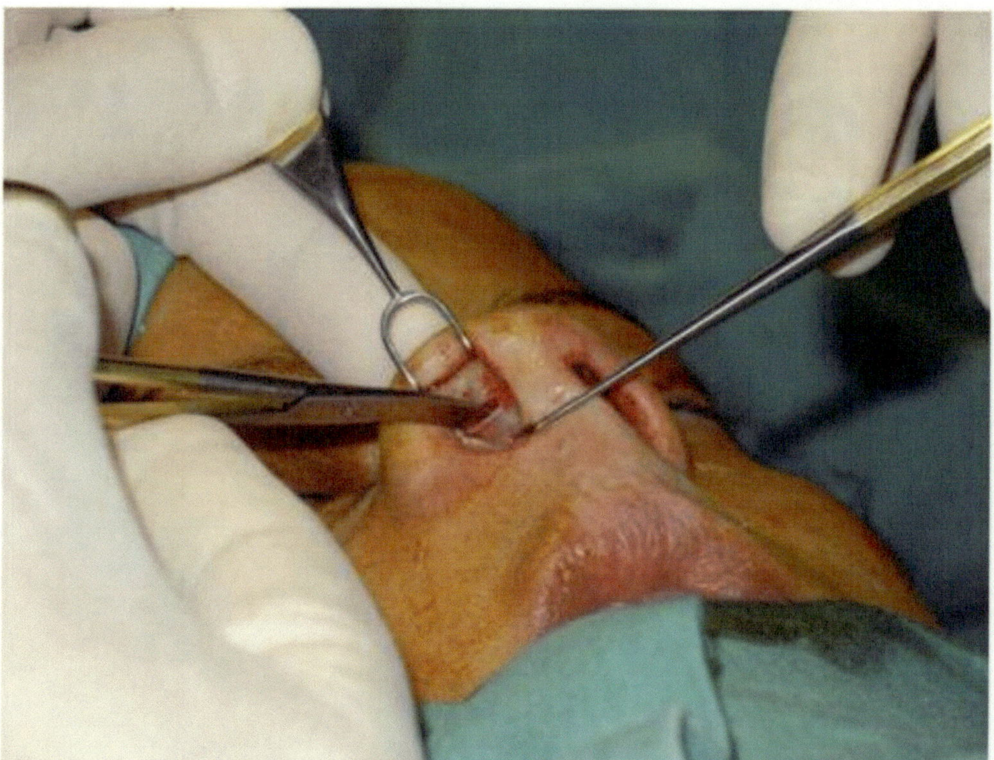

Fig. 2. The cephalic piece of the alar cartilage is dissected and resected

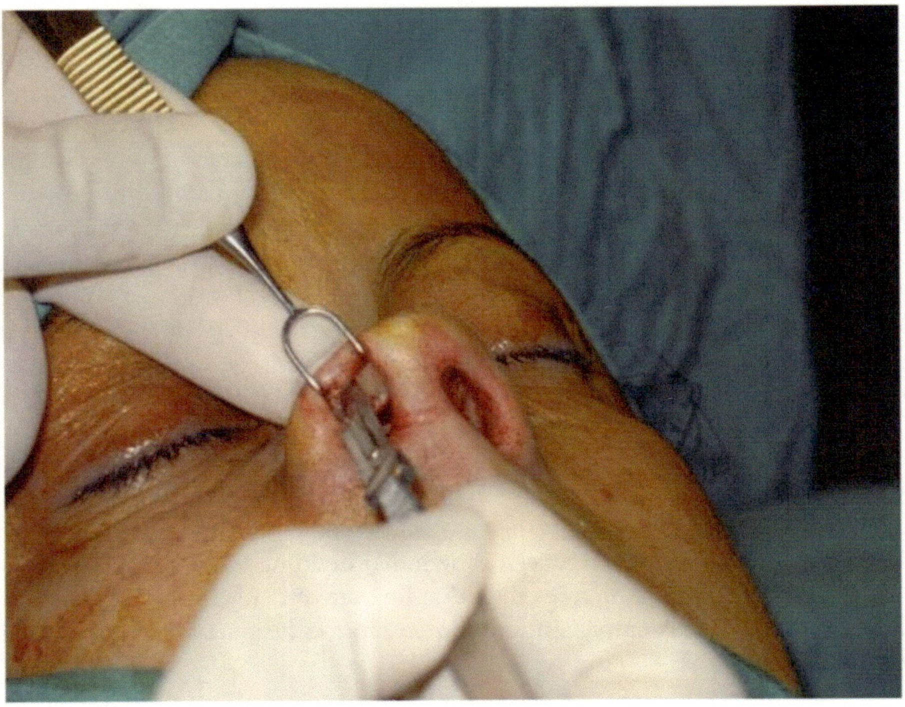

Fig. 3. A marginal incision is made

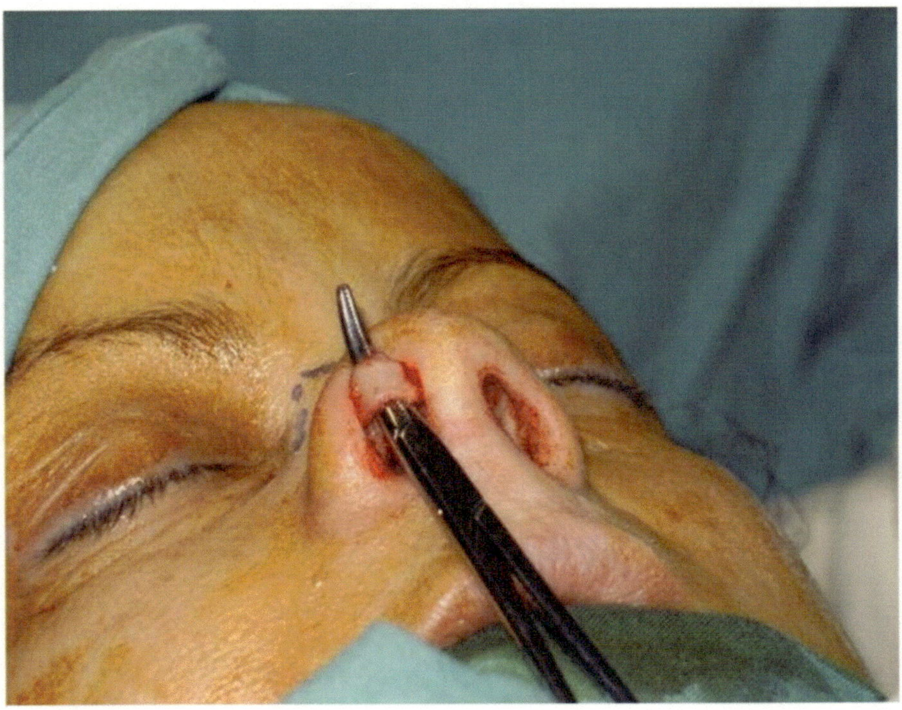

Fig. 4. The remaining alar cartilage is dissected in the non-vestibular side and delivered

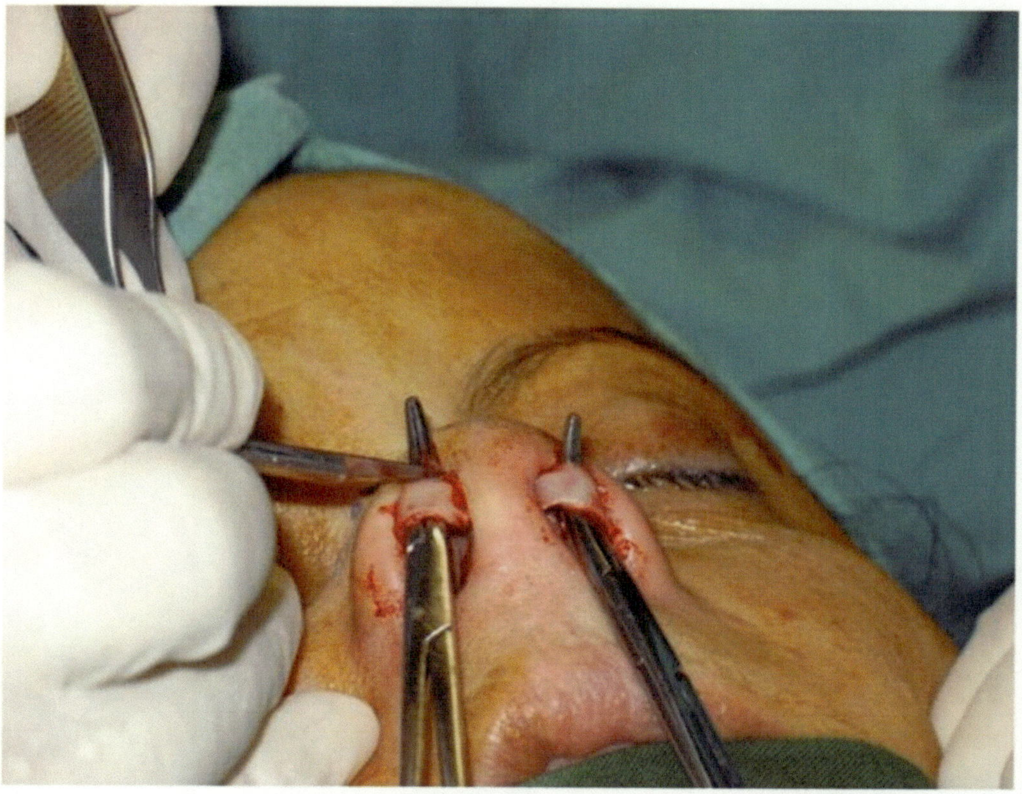

Fig. 5. The remaining alar cartilages are delivered and compared; if necessary, further resection is performed to achieve perfect symmetry or the desired size

We have been using this modification of the delivery approach for several years. In the earlier cases, we used this modified delivery approach only for patients with long alar cartilages (in the cranial-caudal direction) and a wide or bifid nasal tip. We felt that this kind of tip required performing cephalic resection of the alar cartilages plus, if nothing else, a double dome suture. We felt that this modification could make the delivery of long alar cartilages easier and safer, as the cartilage would not be under tension or under a twisting strength at any stage of the procedure. In more recent cases, we have been using this approach for most cases of refinement of the nasal tip, as long as this involved more than just cephalic resection of the alar cartilages. Thus, we have been using the modified delivery approach in almost every case that we would, otherwise, be using the *standard* delivery approach.

The purpose of this modification is combining the advantages of the non-delivery approach with the advantages of the delivery approach in the same procedure, and avoiding an intercartilaginous incision. Thus, the delivery of each alar cartilage is performed in two stages: at the first stage a cephalic piece of the cartilage is resected; at the second stage the remaining alar cartilage is delivered.

The exact amount of cartilage to be resected may be difficult to assess at the first stage, so it is crucial to leave an appropriated sized cartilage caudal to the transcartilaginous incision. At the second stage, after the delivery of the remaining alar cartilages on both sides, these are easily assessed and compared. Further cephalic resection of the alar cartilages may be performed at this stage of the procedure, in order to achieve perfect symmetry or to achieve the desired size of the cartilages.

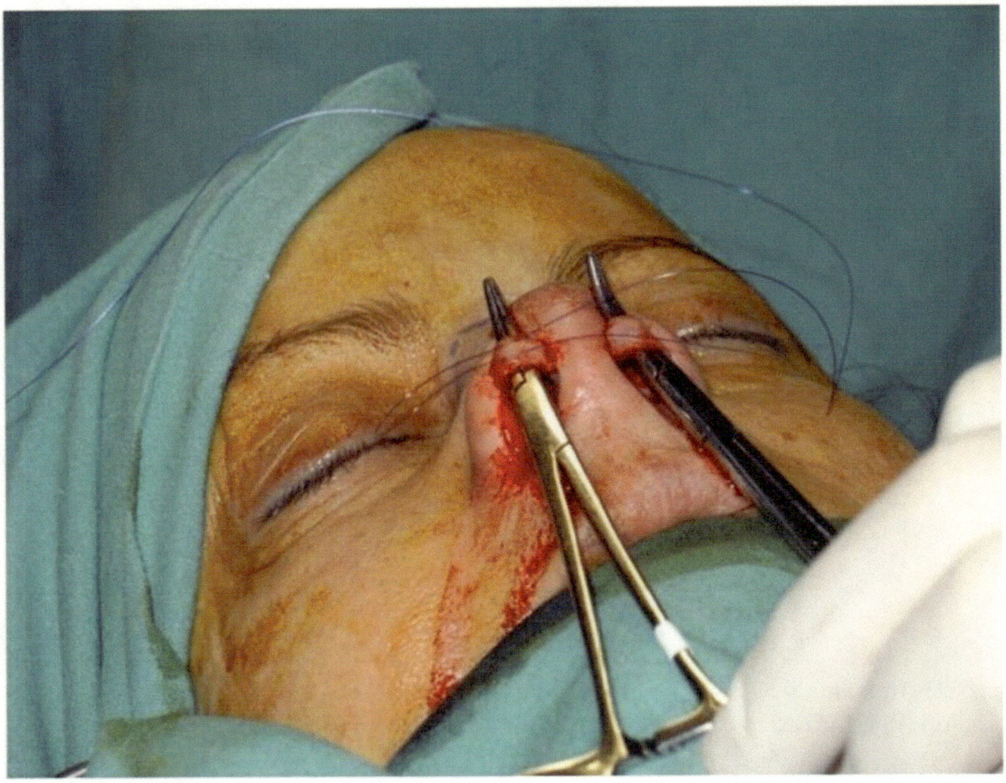

Fig. 6. The other planned manoeuvres, such as domal suturing, are performed

By using first a transcartilaginous incision and then a marginal incision to deliver the alar cartilages, this modified approach combines the reliability of the non-delivery approach with the enhanced exposure of the more powerful delivery approach. By using a transcartilaginous incision instead of an intercartilaginous incision, this modified delivery approach does not promote weakening of one of the *major* tip support mechanisms, the attachment of the upper lateral cartilages to the cephalic margin of the alar cartilages.

4. Conclusion

In rhinoplasty it is often necessary to perform cephalic resection of the alar cartilages to improve tip definition, sometimes combining this procedure with other surgical techniques to the tip, such as single dome or double dome sutures.

The delivery approach may be appropriate to allow all these surgical techniques to be easily executed. However, the intercartilaginous incision usually done for the standard delivery approach may cause a weakening of the tip support by severing the dense collagen fibers at the intercartilaginous region.

A modified delivery approach may be a way to overcome these dangers, facilitating the exposure of the tip cartilages. This modified approach, using a transcartilaginous and a marginal incision, combines the reliability of the non-delivery approach with the enhanced exposure of the delivery approach and avoids the dangers of the intercartilaginous incision.

We have been using this modified delivery approach for several years, and found it particularly useful for patients with long alar cartilages and a wide or bifid nasal tip. We believe that, in this kind of tip, this modified approach is easier to perform and safer to the tip support mechanisms.

5. References

[1] Xavier R. Tip rhinoplasty - a modified delivery approach. *Rhinology* 2009; 47:132-5.

[2] Xavier Rui. A modified delivery approach. In: Shiffman MA, Di Giuseppe A ed. *Advanced Rhinoplasty: Art, Science, and New Clinical Techniques*. Berlin: Springer-Verlag, *in the press*

[3] Tardy ME. Contemporary rhinoplasty: principles and philosophy. In: Behrbohm H, Tardy ME ed. *Essentials of Septorhinoplasty*. Stuttgart-New York: Thieme, 2004: 37-63

[4] Gassner HG, Sherris DA, Friedman O. Rhinology in rhinoplasty. In: Papel ID ed. *Facial Plastic and Reconstructive Surgery*. Stuttgart-New York: Thieme, 2009: 489-506

[5] Han SK, Lee DG, Kim JB, Kim WK. An anatomic study of nasal tip supporting structures. *Ann Plastic Surgery* 2004; 52:134-9.

[6] Han SK, Ko HW, Lee DY, Kim WK. The effect of releasing tip-supporting structures in short-nose correction. *Ann Plastic Surgery* 2005; 54:375-8.

[7] Nolst-Trenité GJ. Basic approaches and techniques in nasal tip surgery. In: Nolst-Trenité GJ ed. *Rhinoplasty 3rd Ed.* The Hague: Kugler Publications, 2005: 87-96

[8] Tardy ME, Toriumi DM, Hecht DA. Philosophy and principles of rhinoplasty. In: Papel ID ed. *Facial Plastic and Reconstructive Surgery*. Stuttgart-New York: Thieme, 2009: 507-528

[9] Nolst-Trenité GJ. Surgery of the nasal tip: intranasal approach. In: Papel ID ed. *Facial Plastic and Reconstructive Surgery*. Stuttgart-New York: Thieme, 2009: 563-576

[10] Kim DW, Toriumi DM. Open structure rhinoplasty. In: Behrbohm H, Tardy ME ed. *Essentials of Septorhinoplasty*. Stuttgart-New York: Thieme, 2004: 117-135

[11] Adamson PA, Litner JA. Open rhinoplasty. In: Papel ID ed. *Facial Plastic and Reconstructive Surgery*. Stuttgart-New York: Thieme, 2009: 529-546

[12] Vuyk HD, Zijlker TD. Open-tip rhinoplasty. In: Nolst-Trenité GJ ed. *Rhinoplasty 3rd Ed.* The Hague: Kugler Publications, 2005: 115-123

[13] Nolst-Trenité GJ, Vinayak BC. External rhinoplasty: the benefits and pitfalls. In: Nolst-Trenité GJ ed. *Rhinoplasty 3rd Ed.* The Hague: Kugler Publications, 2005: 125-141

[14] Whitaker E, Johnson C Jr. The evolution of open structure rhinoplasty. *Arch Facial Plastic Surg*. 2003; 5: 291-300

[15] Farrior E. Dramatic refinement of the nasal tip. *Otolaryngol Clinics of North America.* 1999; 32: 621-636
[16] Oneal R, Beil R Jr, Schlesinger J. Surgical anatomy of the nose. *Otolaryngol Clinics of North America.* 1999; 32: 145-181

Part 3

Reconstructive Challenges

5

Surgical Strategy for Secondary Correction of Unilateral and Bilateral Cleft Lip-Nose Deformities

Norifumi Nakamura
Department of Oral and Maxillofacial Surgery, Field of Maxillofacial Rehabilitation, Kagoshima University Graduate School of Medical and Dental Sciences
Japan

1. Introduction

In the treatment of cleft deformities, restoring the symmetric and natural-shaped nose as well as the symmetric and functional lip is important to allow patients to lead smooth social lives. Recently primary rhinoplasty with presurgical orthopedic treatment for infants with cleft lip and nose has been highlighted (Grayson, et al. 1999), and these techniques have certainly improved nasal deformity and overall symmetry (Nakamura, et al. 2009). However, definitive rhinoplasty may still be necessary as the child grows. Despite recent developments in cleft surgery, the surgical modality for correction of cleft lip-nose deformity that provides a desirable nasal form with long-term stability has not yet been established. Surgeons have attempted cleft lip-nose correction, but they are often frustrated by unsatisfactory results.

A considerable number of surgical modalities for definitive correction of unilateral and bilateral cleft lip-nose deformities have been reported over the past half century. Generally, it is argued that a clear understanding of the associated complex anatomical and pathological abnormalities is required to obtain a desirable nasal form (Shih, et al. 2002). The abnormalities of cleft lip-nose involve all components of the nose, including the facial skeleton, cartilage, muscle, skin, subcutaneous tissue, and mucosal lining. To obtain desirable and stable outcomes, secondary correction of the cleft lip-nose deformity should approach each abnormality in each of the above components. Based on this concept, the author has established the following strategy for secondary cleft lip-nose correction that approaches each anatomical and pathological abnormality causing the main deformities of unilateral and bilateral cleft lip-nose.

2. Treatment strategy for unilateral cleft lip-nose deformity

2.1 Anatomical and pathological characteristics of unilateral cleft lip-nose

Unilateral cleft lip (UCL)-nose deformity includes deviated columella, depressed nasal tip, wide and snub nasal ala, and a flat and V-shaped nostril on the cleft side (Millard, 1976a). The position of the nasal ala on the affected side often dislocates in a downward and distal direction in relation to the inadequately unionized upper lip (Fig. 1A).

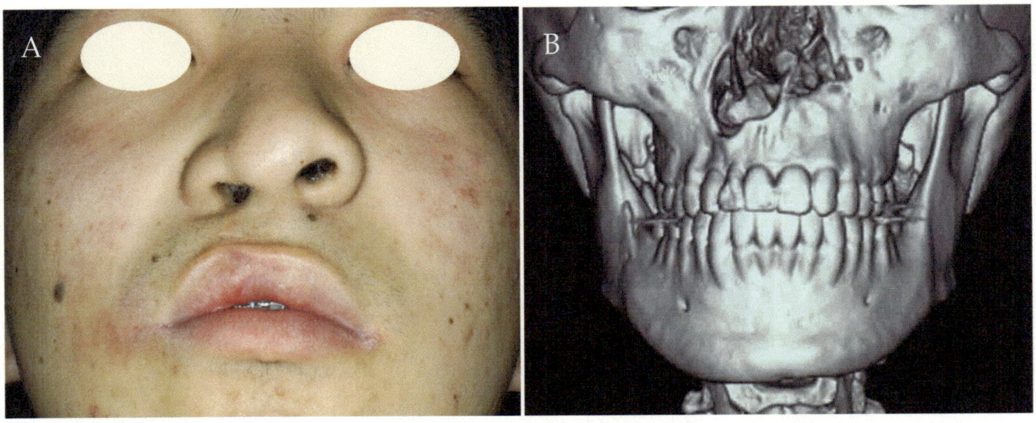

Fig. 1. Facial view (A) and three-dimensional CT finding (B) demonstrating characteristics of UCL-nose deformity

When one considers the characteristics of unilateral cleft lip nose-deformities, the distal, downward, and backward dislocation of the skeletal framework causes all components of the lip and nasal tissue to be malpositioned three-dimensionally on the affected side (Fig. 1A and Fig. 1B). Consequently, the upper and lower lateral cartilages dislocate distally and downwardly, the attachment of the nasalis muscle is malpositioned and skin at the nostril rim forms a web. Additionally, excessive stress over the nasal tip and dorsum causes growth disturbances of the septal cartilage, resulting in a short columella and flared nasal tip on the affected side.

To facilitate an understanding of these abnormalities, the unilateral cleft lip-nose can be thought to be like a house built on a slope (Fig. 2). The center pole corresponds to the nasal septum, the roof is the lower lateral cartilage and skin, the lateral pillar is the vestibule, and the ground is the maxillary bone. In the normal nose, the ground is flat and the house can stand upright (Fig. 2A), but in the unilateral cleft lip-nose, the house is on a slope and the pole and roof incline toward the downward side (Fig. 2B). To create a straight house on a slope, the center pole must stand upright in the center of the face, the pillar should be expanded and roof should be lifted upward (Fig. 2C).

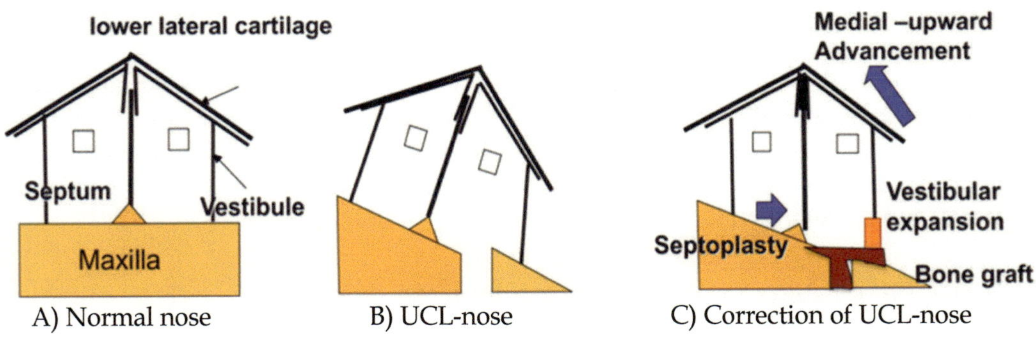

Fig. 2. Anatomical and pathologic abnormalities of UCL-nose; normal nose (A), UCL-nose (B), and correction of UCL-nose (C) *(Modified from Nakamura, Jpn J Oral Maxillofac Surg 2010)*

Table 1 demonstrates the treatment strategy for unilateral cleft lip-nose, showing an approach to each anatomical and pathological abnormality causing the main deformities of unilateral cleft lip-nose: deviated columella, depressed and deviated nasal tip, wide and snub nasal ala, and flat and V-shaped nonstril on the cleft side (Table 1). Therefore, the author's secondary correction involves open rhinoplasty, septoplasty, repositioning of the lower lateral cartilage, medial and upward advancement of the lip and nose components; the nasal vestibular tissues, the nasal ala, nasalis muscle, and the upper part of the lip including orbicular oris muscle, and nasal vestibular expansion with or without bone graft (Fig. 2C).

nasal deformities	anatomical pathological abnormalities	surgical procedures in the secondary correction
● deviated columella	· deviation of midline of maxilla · deviated septal cartilage	· dissection around anterior nasal spine · reposition of inferior base of septal cartilage, if necessary
● depressed and deviated nasal tip	· distally and downwardly dislocated lower lateral cartilage on the cleft side · growth disturbances of septal cartilage	· freeing and repositioning of lower lateral cartilage by overlapping on the upper lateral cartilage · caudal septal extension graft
● wide and snub nasal ala on cleft side	· retropositioned anterior maxillary wall · dislocation of the attachment of nasalis muscle	· secondary bone graft, if necessary · supraperiosteal dissection around piriform margin · reposition of the nasalis muscle by medial-upward advancement of nasolabial components
● flat and V-shaped nostril	· webbing of the rim skin · shortage of the nasal vestibular lining · disconnection of orbicularis oris muscle	· bilaterally symmetric reverse-U incision · expansion of the nasal vestibule · overlapped suturing of orbicularis oris muscle

Table 1. Nasal deformity and treatment strategy for unilateral cleft lip-nose *(Modified form Nakamura, et al. J Oral Maxillofac Surg 2010)*

2.2 Surgical procedures for correction of unilateral cleft lip-nose deformities (Fig. 3 and Fig. 4)

1. Open rhinoplasty is applied according to the bilateral reverse-U incision and transcolumellar incision. A reverse-U incision is made on the outer skin slightly above the nostril rim in order to lengthen the upper columella on the affected side (Fig. 3A and Fig. 4A). The distal ends of the incision are extended into the nostril and connected to the back cut incision along the nasal vestibule. The lower end of the back cut incision is extended to the nasal floor and to the white lip along previous surgical scars, when simultaneous correction of upper lip deformity is necessary.
2. Through the oral and nasal vestibular incision, supraperiosteal dissection surrounding the piriform margin is performed on the affected side. This dissection provides 3D movement of the nasal alar base and enables the medial-upward advancement of the nasolabial components.
3. Deviation of the columellar base is corrected by supraperiosteal dissection around the anterior nasal spine through the oral vestibular incision. When the base of the nasal septum is severely deviated, the inferior edge of the septal cartilage is excised to allow repositioning to the midline, and then it is secured to the small hole made at the piriform bottom using a 4-0 Nylon thread (Fig. 4B and Fig. 5).
4. Reflecting the nose tip skin, the malpositioned lower lateral alar cartilage is exposed from both the nasal skin and lining mucosa, and the distal ends of the lateral crura are freed from the surrounding tissue (Fig. 3B and Fig. 4C). Since the corrected cartilage is often insufficiently supported, a small, square cartilaginous strut approximately 8 - 10 mm x 15 mm is taken from the lower part of the nasal septum, and transferred to the

anterior edge of the nasal septum; a caudal septal extension graft (Fig. 4D and Fig. 5). When the growth of the nasal septum is too underdeveloped, free auricular cartilage is used for a caudal septal extension graft. The medial crus of the lower lateral cartilage on the affected side is repositioned in a slightly overlapped position on the upper lateral cartilage and fixed symmetrically to the caudal septal extension graft using a 6-0 Nylon thread (Fig. 4E and Fig. 5B).

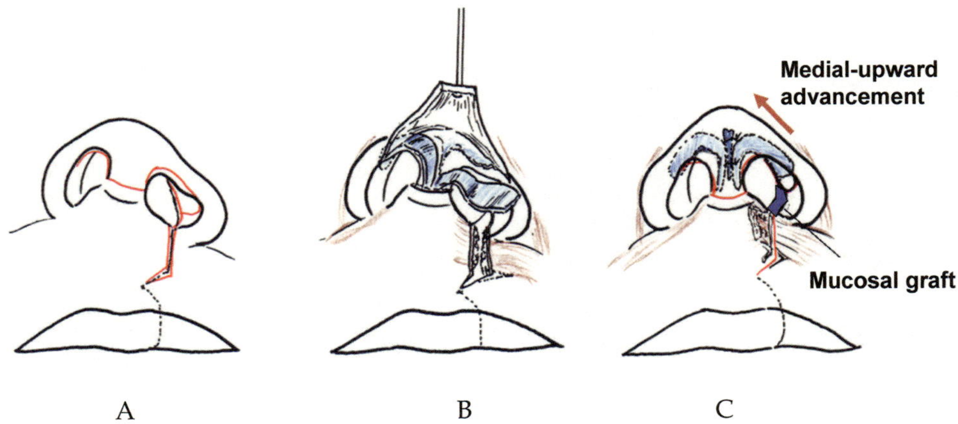

Fig. 3. Surgical procedures for correction of unilateral cleft lip-nose deformity *(Nakamura, et al. J Oral Maxillofac Surg 2010)*

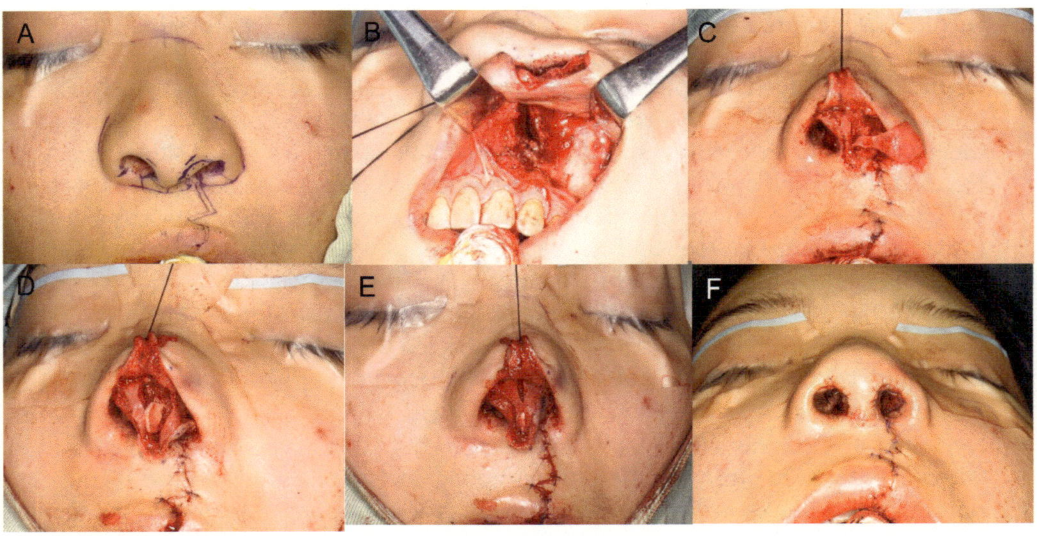

Fig. 4. Step-by-step procedures for correction of unilateral cleft lip-nose deformity *(Nakamura, et al. J Oral Maxillofac Surg 2010)*

5. After the nasal tip skin is redraped, the nasal lining is advanced medially and upwardly to cover the nostril dome (Fig. 3C). The excess skin at the nostril rim on the cleft side is also reflected and pushbacked into the canopy of the nostril dome. The defect of lining at the nasal vestibule caused by the above advancement is then covered by a free

mucosal graft donated from the buccal area or covered by the tissue advanced from the bottom of the nasal floor (Fig. 3C)

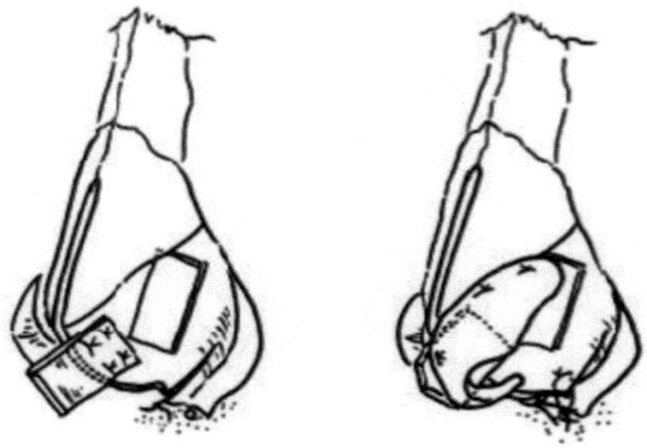

A B

Fig. 5. Reposition of the lower lateral cartilage with a caudal septal extension graft
(Nakamura, et al. J Oral Maxillofac Surg 2010)

6. When simultaneous correction of upper lip deformity is carried out, the nasalis muscle and the orbicularis oris muscle are separated along the previous scar. After dissecting these muscles from the maxillary wall, the distal bundle of nasalis muscle is then connected to the periosteum surrounding the anterior nasal spine, and the medial and distal bundles of orbicularis oris muscle are connected in an overlapping manner using a mattress suture technique (Fig. 3C). At the end of surgery, subcutaneous and cutaneous suturing is carefully performed (Fig. 4F).

2.3 Pre- and postoperative views and three-dimensional observation of patients treated for unilateral cleft lip-nose deformity

Pre- and postoperative photos and the three-dimensional (3D) color images of the patients are demonstrated in figure 6 and figure 7. Preoperative views demonstrate the deviated nasal tip, asymmetric and wide peak of the nasal hump and obviously small and flat nasal ala on the affected side. The nostril on the affected side is flatter than that on the healthy side in both patients. 3D color images indicate asymmetry of the alar groove and nasal tip more visually. The top of the alar groove on the cleft side is dislocated distally and downwardly resulting in a small snub ala.

Postoperative photos and 3D color images in the frontal and basal views demonstrate symmetric nasal forms. The nasal tip projection is recovered in the center of the face and the height and the appropriate contour of the nasal ala groove on the cleft side are improved satisfactorily. The nostril demonstrates a symmetric and desirable form postoperatively. The contour between the columella and the upper lip in the lateral view appears quite natural.

The author has performed secondary treatment of unilateral cleft lip-nose on more than 50 patients, and there have not been any serious complications such as necrosis of the skin flap, infection, or airway obstruction, nor any obvious scars or deformities involving the upper lip and/or columellar base in any patient.

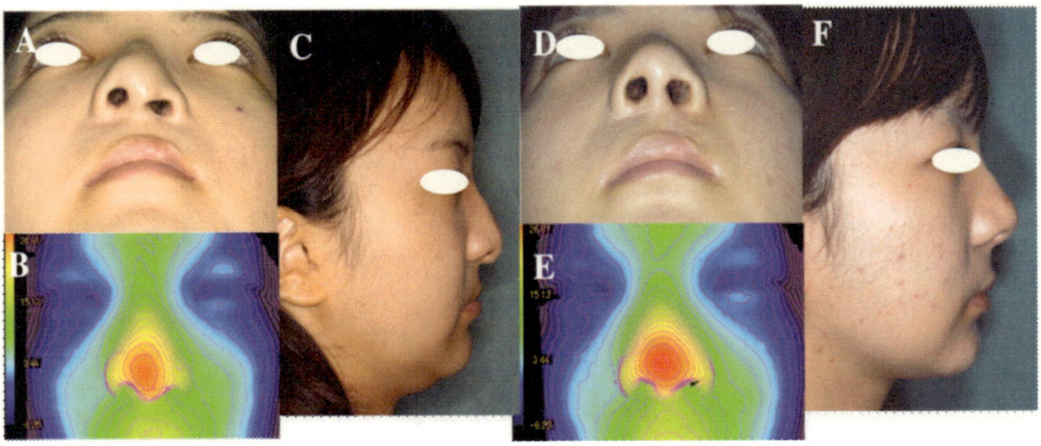

Fig. 6. Pre- and postoperative nasal views and 3D images of a female with UCLP whose correction is shown in figure 4. *(Nakamura, et al. J Oral Maxillofac Sug 2010)*

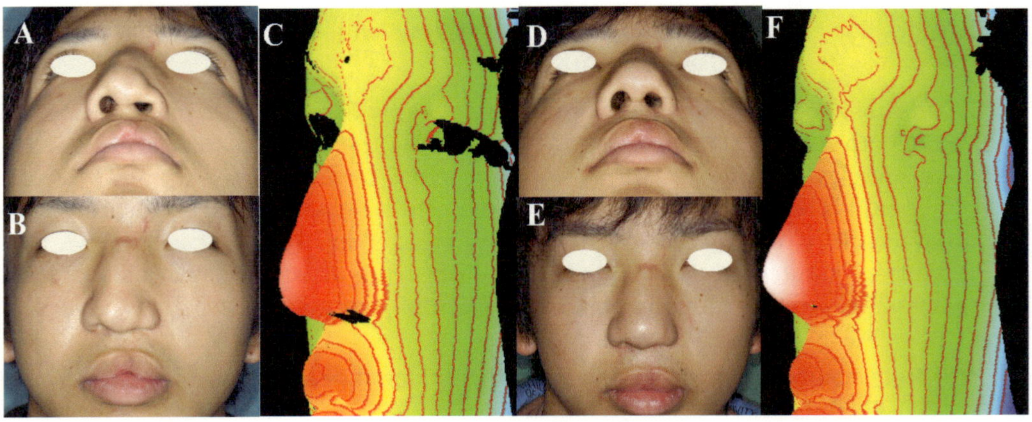

Fig. 7. Pre- and postoperative nasal views and 3D images of a male with UCLP

3. Treatment of strategy for bilateral cleft lip-nose deformity

3.1 Anatomical and pathological characteristics of bilateral cleft lip-nose

Bilateral cleft lip (BCL)-nose deformity is characterized mainly by a columella with varying degrees of shortness, a depressed nasal tip, bilateral dislocation of the alar cartilage, and eversion of the alar bases (Fig. 8)(Millard, 1976b). When one considers the characteristics of bilateral cleft lip-nose, the deformities might be basically considered the combined characteristics of a unilateral cleft lip-nose on both sides, including varying degrees of anterior overgrowth of the premaxilla. Due to the lateral, downward, and backward dislocation of the bilateral skeletal framework, all components of the lip and nasal tissues are also malpositioned three dimensionally. Consequently, the attachment of the nasal muscle is malpositioned, bilateral major alar cartilages are separated distally and downwardly, and nostril rim skin forms a web. Additionally, the excessive stress over the nasal tip and dorsum causes growth disturbances of the septal cartilage, resulting in a short columella and flared nasal tip. Therefore, it is more physiological to advance all nasal tip components medially and upwardly after dissecting free from the dislocated anterior maxillary wall, as in unilateral cleft lip-nose correction, and to supply lateral tissue to the columella rather than the upper lip.

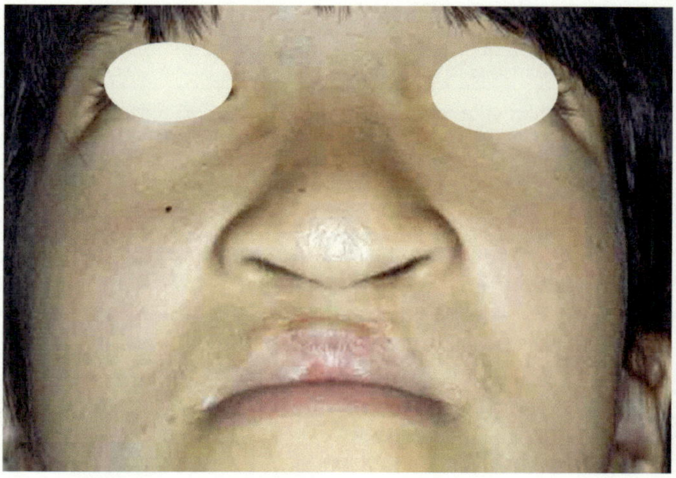

Fig. 8. Characteristics of BCL-nose deformity

The anatomical and pathological abnormality of the bilateral cleft lip-nose can also explained by the metaphor of a house compressed by stress (Fig. 9). The basic principle is the same as that for the unilateral cleft lip-nose. To create a normal form, the center pole in the house should be extended at the center, and the roof advanced upwardly, and then the pillar on each side should be extended. Most important, the stress should be removed, which corresponds to pulling on the nasal tip due the shortage of columellar skin.

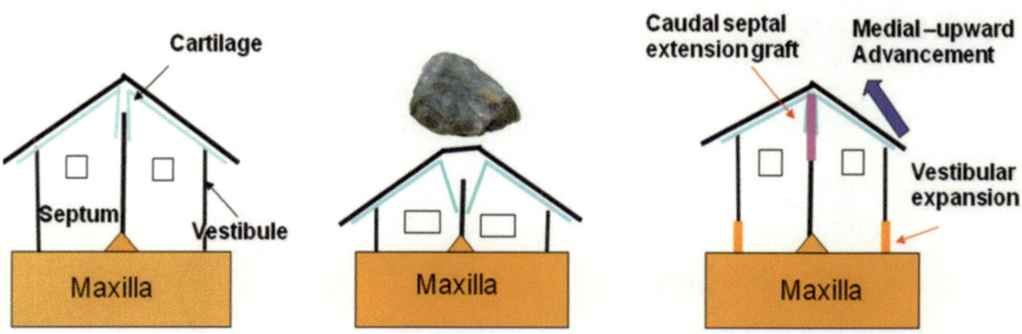

Fig. 9. Anatomical and pathologic abnormality of BCL-nose; normal nose (A), BCL-nose (B), and correction of BCL-nose (C)

The author has established a surgical strategy based on the principle that the ideal technique for secondary treatment of bilateral cleft lip-nose deformity should minimize damage to either or both the upper and lower lip tissue as shown in Table 2. This strategy also approaches each anatomical and pathological abnormality that causes the main deformities of the bilateral cleft lip-nose: short columella, flat and flared nasal tip, wide and snub nasal alar, and flat and V-shaped nostril (Table 2). Therefore, the author's secondary correction involves open rhinoplasty, repositioning of the lower lateral cartilages, a caudal septal extension graft, medial and upward advancement of the lip and nose components, nasal vestibular expansion, and columella lengthening using a nostril rim rotation flap, if necessary.

nasal deformities	anatomical pathological anomalies	surgical procedures in the secondary correction
● short columella	･shortage of the columellar skin ･tightness of the subcutaneous tissue in the columella	･bilateral reverse-U incision ･nostril rim skin rotation flap, if necessary ･V-Y elongation of the fibrous tissue
● flat and flared nasal tip	･growth disturbance of septal cartilage ･lateral and downward dislocation of lower lateral cartilage ･thin skin envelope of the nasal tip	･caudal septal extension graft ･freeing and reposition of lower lateral cartilage by overlapping on the upper lateral cartilage ･molding up the fibrous tissue on the nasal tip
● wide and snub nasal ala	･dislocation of attachment of nasal muscle	･supraperiosteal dissection around piriform margin ･reposition of nasal muscle by the medial and upper advancement of nasal alar component
● flat and V-shaped nostril	･webbing of the rim skin ･shortage of nasal vestibular lining ･disconnection of orbicular oris muscle	･bilateral reverse-U incision ･free mucosal graft in the nasal vestibule ･reposition of orbicularis oris muscle

Table 2. Nasal deformity and treatment strategy for bilateral cleft lip-nose *(Modified from Nakamura, et al. J Cranio-Maxillofac Surg 2011)*

3.2 Surgical procedures for correction of bilateral cleft lip-nose deformities (Fig. 10 and Fig. 11)

1. Open rhinoplasty is applied according to the bilateral reverse U incision and transcolumellar incision, but rim incisions on the bilateral side are made on the outer skin slightly above the nostril rim in order to lengthen the upper columella. The distal ends of the incision are extended into the nostril and connected to the back cut incision along the posterior edge of the nasal vestibule (Fig. 10A and Fig. 11A).

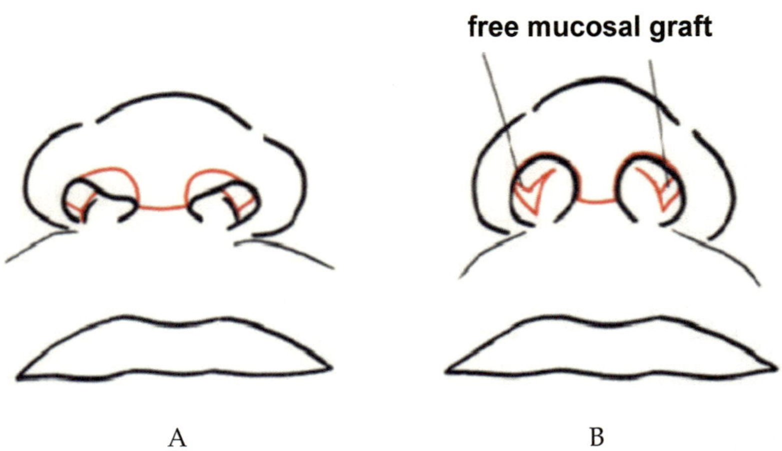

Fig. 10. Surgical procedures for correction of bilateral cleft lip-nose deformity *(Nakamura, et al. J Cranio-Maxillofac Surg 2011)*

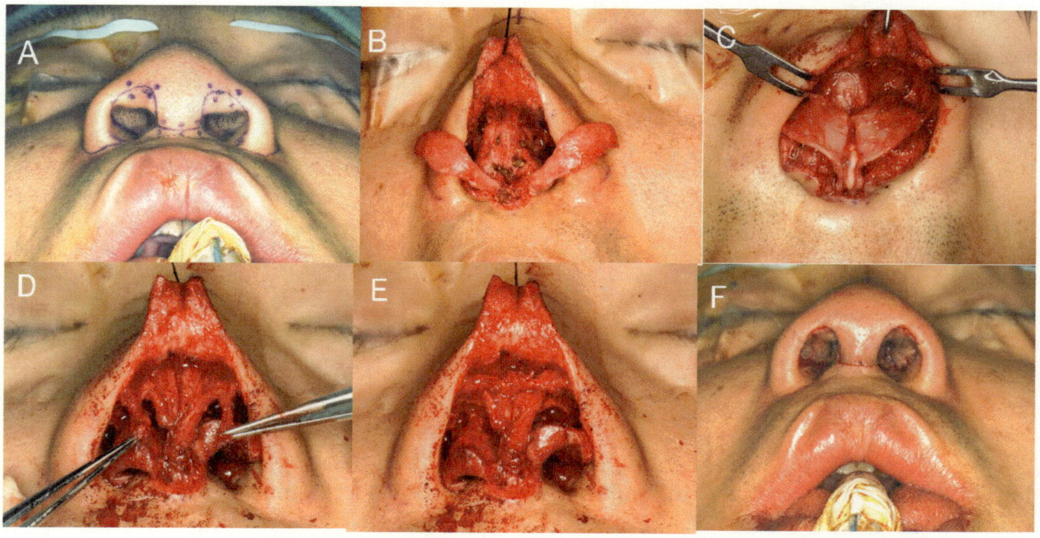

Fig. 11. Step-by-step procedures for correction of bilateral cleft lip-nose deformity
(Nakamura, et al. J Cranio-Maxillofac Surg 2011)

2. Through oral and nasal vestibular incision, supraperiosteal dissection surrounding the piriform margin and lower border of the upper lateral cartilage is performed. These dissections allow repositioning of the nasalis muscle at an adequate position on the anterior maxillary wall and facilitate 3D medial-upward-frontal advancement of the nasal alar base (Fig. 10B).
3. Reflecting the nose tip skin, the malpositioned lower lateral cartilages are exposed from both the nasal skin and lining mucosa, and the distal ends of the lateral crura are freed from the upper lateral cartilages (Fig. 11B). Cartilaginous strut is then transferred to the anterior edge of the nasal septum to produce nasal tip projection. Medial crura of the bilateral lower lateral cartilages are repositioned in a slightly overlapped position on the upper lateral cartilage and fixed to the caudal septal extension graft symmetrically by a 6-0 Nylon thread (Fig. 11C). When the growth of the nasal septum is too underdeveloped to use a cartilaginous graft, free auricular cartilage is transferred to the nasal tip.
4. To resolve the tightness of the skin envelope that often causes the collapse of the caudal septal extension graft, subcutaneous fibrous tissue is widely dissected around the nasal tip, and then elongated by the V-Y method at the columellar base. To produce the nasal tip projection, the lateral parts of the subcutaneous fibrous tissue are dissected vertically and molded on the nasal tip (Fig. 11D and E). When the nasal tip skin is redraped and skin is insufficient to cover the base of columella due to the improved nasal projection, inferiorly based small pedicle flaps (Ohishi, et al. 1996) are made from the rim skin below the incision and rotated medially into the raw area of the columellar base (Fig. 12).
5. After repositioning the lower lateral cartilage, the nasal lining tissue is advanced medially and upwardly to cover the nostril dome. The defects of lining at the nasal vestibule caused by the upward advancement of the alar component are then covered by a free mucosal graft donated from the buccal area (Fig. 10B and Fig. 12C).
6. At the end of the operation, subcutaneous and cutaneous suturing is carefully performed (Fig. 11F), and sponge tube nasal stent is applied for 1 week postoperatively.

A silicon nostril retainer (Koken Co., Tokyo, Japan) is then placed and kept in situ for at least 3 months postoperatively.

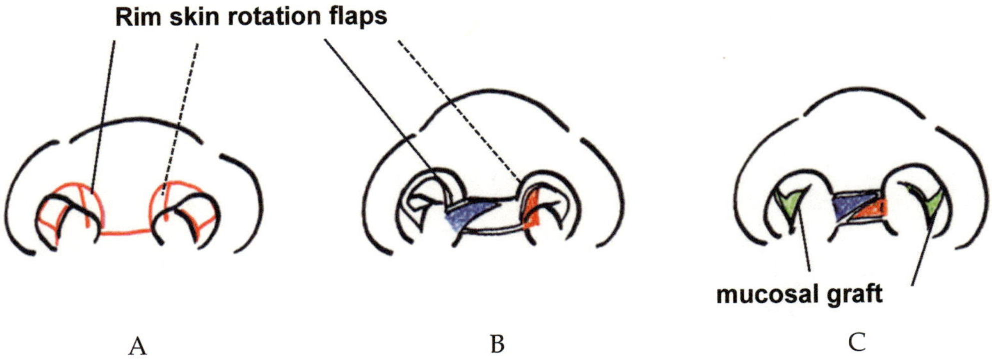

Fig. 12. Inferiorly based rim skin rotation flap for columella lengthening *(Nakamura, et al. J Cranio-Maxillofac Surg 2011)*

3.3 Pre- and postoperative views and three-dimensional observation of patients treated for bilateral cleft lip-nose deformity

Pre- and postoperative views and 3D color images of patients treated for bilateral cleft lip-nose deformity are shown in figure 13 and figure 14. Preoperative photos and 3D images demonstrate the short columella and flattened nasal tip in both patients. The frontal and oblique 3D color images indicate wide peaked nasal tip demonstrating a pseudo nasal hump visually. Bilateral nasal alas are almost symmetric but the nasal alar grooves on both sides are small demonstrating snub forms.

Postoperative photos and 3D color images demonstrate symmetric nasal forms with adequately projected nasal tip by successful columella lengthening in both patients. The appropriate contours of the nasal ala groove on both sides are symmetrically expanded resulting in a natural transition from nasal tip to ala.

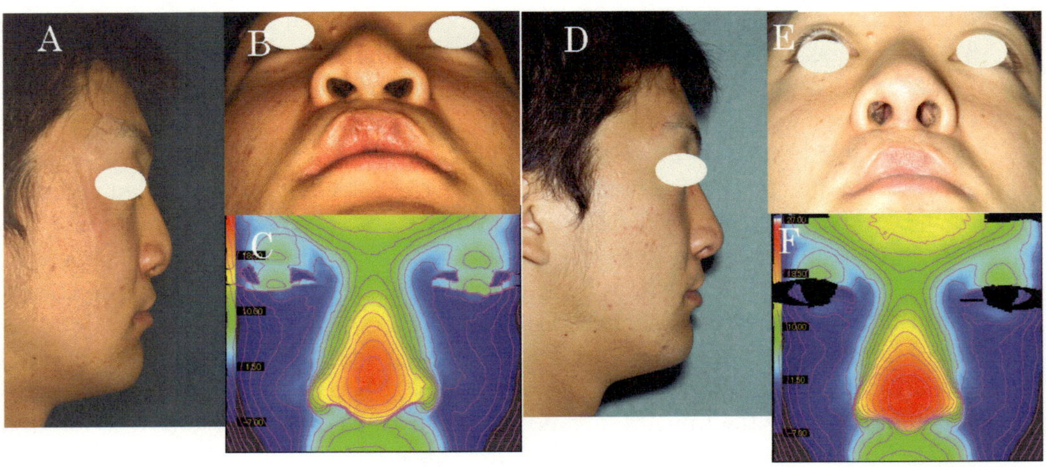

Fig. 13. Pre- and postoperative nasal views and 3D images of a male with BCLP whose correction is shown in figure 11 *(Nakamura, et al. J Cranio-Maxillofac Surg 2011)*

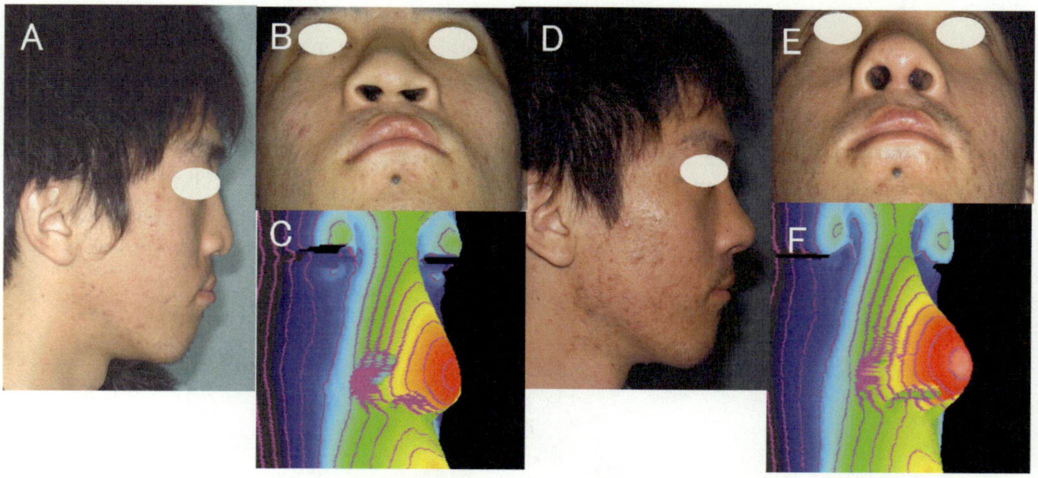

Fig. 14. Pre- and postoperative nasal views and 3D images of a male with BCLP *(Modified from Nakamura, et al. J Cranio-Maxillofac Surg 2011)*

The author has performed secondary treatment of bilateral cleft lip-nose using these techniques on more than 20 patients. There were no wide necroses of the skin flap, infection, airway obstruction, nor any obvious scars or deformities in the upper lip and/or columellar base in any patient. A small area of necrosis at the tip of the nostril rim rotation flap was observed in some patients, and the most persistent postoperative problem was contraction of large free mucosal graft in the vestibular lining.

4. Benefits and limitations of the author's correction for unilateral and bilateral cleft lip-nose

Regarding the treatment of unilateral cleft lip-nose, several benefits have been demonstrated from our previous data of pre- and postoperative 3D observations (Okawachi, et al. 2011). First, repositioning of the open reduction of the lower lateral cartilage with slight overlapping of the upper lateral cartilage with the caudal septal extension graft can provide a symmetric and projected nasal tip form. Second, repositioning of the septal cartilage through an oral vestibular incision recovers the nasal midline in half of the nose. Third, medial-upward advancement of the nasolabial components with vestibular expansion repositions the malattached nasalis muscles on the affected side and provides a symmetric and expanded nasal alar form.

One of the most serious problems of the nose is a deviated and depressed nasal tip. There are numerous modalities for unilateral nasal tip correction, and many previous reports mainly focused on correction of the nasal repositioning, and molding (Spira, et al. 1970, Millard, 1976a, Salyer, 1992). In the author's nose correction procedures, nasal tip correction is achieved by repositioning of the lower lateral cartilage through open rhinoplasty and a caudal septal extension graft, and these procedures are the same as those previously reported (Byrd, et al. 1997, Shih, et al. 2002, Rettinger, et al. 2002). For a caudal septal extension graft, the author favors septal cartilage donated from the lower part of the nasal septum because of its straight form and hardness, but when the growth of the nasal septum is too underdeveloped, free auricular cartilage is used. During surgery the affected lower lateral cartilage is carefully repositioned to a symmetric position to avoid an overprojected nose by measuring the nasolabial angle during surgery. Since the nasolabial angle in Japanese adults (95-100°) is smaller than that of Caucasians (90-110°) (Ozumi, 2006), excessive projection of the nasal tip provides an undesirable nose form. Therefore, the author has prepared an original metal scale to measure the nasolabial angle during the surgery. The metal scale had sample corners with angles of 90°, 100°, 110°, 120°, and 130° (Fig. 15). When the angle was greater than the Japanese average, the position of the strut graft can be changed during surgery; consequently an undesirable overprojection of the nasal tip can be avoided.

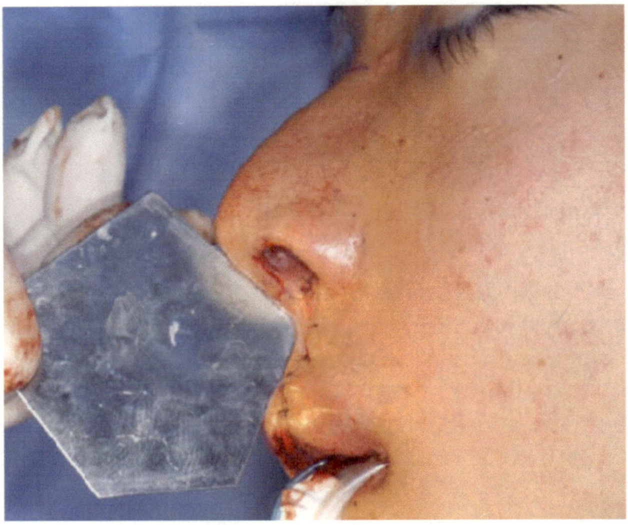

Fig. 15. Original metal scale for measuring nasolabial angle intraoperatively *(Nakamura, et al. J Oral Maxillofac Surg 2010)*

Another conspicuous deformity of unilateral cleft lip-nose is the small and deviated nasal ala on the affected side. Even though correction of the nasal tip projection is fully achieved, asymmetric and poorly expanded nasal ala is often persistent in patients with unilateral cleft lip. It is considered that the nasal alar form is affected by not only alar cartilage but also anomalies of the surrounding tissues, such as tightness of the skin envelope, dislocated nasalis muscle, and insufficient vestibular lining. Therefore, it is essential to advance the nasal components upwardly repositioning the nasalis muscles as well as reconstruct the nasal cartilages for treatment of a small ala. Vestibular expansion also ensures prevention of postoperative collapse of the support of the lower lateral cartilage. Additionally, the improvement of the maxillary platform by bone graft is important to correct the dislocated nasal ala. The author performs secondary bone graft in the alveolar cleft and anterior surface of the piriform margin at approximately 9-11 years of age. Furthermore, when backward dislocation of the nasal alar base is remarkable at the secondary correction of nose, a veneer graft of cortical bone donated from the anterior edge of the mandibular ramus is used to mold the area around the piriform margin. However, in the author's experience, a medial and upward advancement of nasolabial components and reposition of the nasalis muscle is more effective than bone graft to correct a small nasal ala on the affected nose.

Regarding secondary treatment of bilateral cleft lip-nose, there have been a considerable number of surgical modalities reported for bilateral cleft lip-nose correction, and many of these methods have focused on elongation of the short columella by a forked-flap technique (Millard, 1976b), Cronin's (1958) and Converse's (1957) method, and advancement of the prolabium into the columella in combination with an Abbe flap (Yonehara et al, 2008). For correction of short columellar skin, we perform bilateral reverse-U incision when the skin shortage is slight or mild, and a nostril rim skin rotation flap is combined when the columella is extremely short (Ohishi, et al, 1996). V-Y elongation of the fibrous tissue in the columellar base is also combined because tension from this often disturbs the nasal tip projection. This technique has several advantages: 1) the flap utilizes the web skin below the incision of the nostril rim; 2) there is no tissue supply needed and no additional scar on the upper lip as a result; and 3) good color matching and the natural contour at the columella-labial junction are possible and no conspicuous scar is observed on the columellar base. Furthermore, 4) the surgical procedure for columella lengthening can be selected from bilateral reverse-U incision alone or in combination with nostril rim skin flap, depending on the severity of the shortage of columellar skin (Nakamura, et al. 2011). Disadvantages of this technique include the fragility and relatively small size of the nostril skin flap. A small area of necrosis at the tip of the nostril rim rotation flap resulting in postoperative scar contraction of the flap tends to create an uneven contour of columella.

One of the challenges in augmentation rhinoplasty is the tissue contracture that has occurred prior to framework surgery, especially in bilateral cleft lip-nose. Tightness of the skin envelope often limits a space for repositioning the lower lateral cartilage and molding the soft tissues around the nasal tip area, even the wide nasal undermining is carried out. To resolve this problem, the author carefully performs nasal undermining along a single plane beyond the lower part of the upper lateral cartilage and piriform margin that enables nasal tissue advancement providing reattachment of the nasalis muscles in a higher position on the anterior maxillary wall. When these procedures are completed, sufficient enlargement of the skin envelop for nasal tip augmentation that is tolerated without inducing or attenuation of the overlying skin can be achieved.

Complications resulting from our correction of bilateral cleft lip-nose deformity were not serious, but the most persistent postoperative problem was postoperative contraction of large free mucosal graft in the vestibular lining. Therefore, a sufficient supply for vestibular lining is thought to be required, and when lip repair is accompanied, it is more reliable to advance the tissue at the nostril floor upwardly to close the defects of the vestibular lining in order to avoid the risk of scar contraction of the grafted tissue. Additionally, the use of vasuclularized mucosal flaps that may be harvested from the nasal interior (e.g. from septum, turbinates, nasal floor, etc.) might be less prone to contracture than the free mucosal graft (Burget and Menick, 1989). Longer application of the nasal stent will be also useful to maintain the nasal form.

5. Conclusion

Finally, the author concludes that our surgical strategy for secondary correction of unilateral and bilateral cleft lip-nose is useful for providing satisfactory results, producing symmetric and projected nasal tip and ala without damaging the upper lip tissue for Asian patients. This approach may also be useful in Caucasian patients, when the columella is not too short. Repositioning of the nasalis muscle and sufficient expansion of the nasal vestibule as well as reconstruction of the nasal cartilage are important for correction of unilateral and bilateral cleft lip-nose deformity.

6. References

Burget GC and Menick FJ: Nasal support and lining: The marrige of beauty and blood supply. *Plast Reconstr Surg* 84:189, 1989.

Byrd HS, Andochick S, Copit S, Waltom KG: Septal extension grafts: A method of controlling tip projection shape. *Plast Reconstr Surg* 100:999, 1997.

Converse JM: Corrective surgery of the nasal tip. *Laryngoscope* 67:16, 1957.

Cronin TD: Lengthening columella by use of skin from nasal floor and alae. *Plast Reconstr Surg* 21:417, 1958.

Grayson BH, Santiago PE, Brecht LE, Cutting CB: Presurgical nasoalveolar molding in infants with cleft lip and palate. *Cleft Palate-Craniofac J* 36:486, 1999.

Millard DR Jr: The anatomy of the secondary deformity of the unilateral cleft lip nose. In: *Cleft Craft. The evolution of its surgery.* Vol. I, The Unilateral Deformities. Boston, Little, Brown and Company, 1976a, p629.

Millard DR Jr: The anatomy of the secondary bilateral nasal deformity. In: *Cleft Craft. The evolution of its surgery.* Vol. II, The Bilateral and Rare Deformities. Boston: Little, Brown and Company 1976b, P477.

Nakamura N, Sasaguri M, Nozoe E, Nishihara K, Hasegawa H, Nakamura S: Postoperative nasal forms after presurgical nasoalveolar molding followed by medial-upward advancement of the nasolabial components with vestibular expansion for children with unilateral complete cleft lip and palate. *J Oral Maxillofac Surg* 67:2222, 2009.

Nakamura N, Okawachi T, Nishihara K, Hirahara N, Nozoe E: Surgical technique for secondary correction of unilateral cleft lip nose deformity –Clinical and three dimensional observations of pre- and postoperative nasal forms-. *J Oral Maxillofac Surg* 68:2248, 2010.

Nakamura N: Minimally invase treatment of unilateral cleft lip nose deformity by pesurgical nasoalveolar molding followed by medial-upward advancement of nasolabial components (*in Japanese with English abstract*). *Jpn J Oral Maxillofac Surg* 56:618, 2010.

Nakamura N, Sasaguri M, Okawachi T, Nishihara K, Nozoe E: Secondary correction of bilateral cleft lip nose deformity –clinical and three-dimensional observations on pre- and postoperative outcomes-. *J Cranio-Maxillofacial Surg* 39:305, 2011.

Ohishi M, Nakamura N, Yoshikawa H, Goto K, Honda Y: A new method of columella lengthening for correction of cleft lip nose deformity (Abstract). *J Cranio-Maxillofac Surg* 24:84, 1996.

Okawachi T, Nozoe E, Nishihara K, Nakamura N: 3-Dimensinal analyses of outcomes following secondary treatment of unilateral cleft lip nose deformity. *J Oral Maxillofac Surg* 69:322, 2011.

Ozumi K: Aesthetic surgery of the nasal tip and columella (*in Japanese with English abstract*). Keisei Geka 49:663, 2006.

Rettinger G, O'Connell M: The nasal base in cleft lip rhinoplasty. *Facial Plast Surg* 18:165, 2002.

Salyer, KE: Early and late treatment of unilateral cleft nasal deformity. *Cleft Palate-Craniofac J* 29:556, 1992.

Shih CW, Sykes JM: Correction of the cleft-lip nasal deformity. *Facial Plast Surg* 18:253, 2002.

Spira M, Hardy SB, Gerow FJ: Correction of nasal deformities accompanying unilateral cleft lip. *Cleft Palate J* 7:112, 1970.

Yonehara Y, Mori Y, Chikazu D, Saijo H, Takato T: Secondary correction of bilateral cleft lip and nasal deformity by simultaneous placement of an Abbe flap, septal cartilage graft and cantilevered iliac bone graft. *J Oral Maxillofac Surg* 66:581, 2008.

6

Thin Nasal Shell

Paul O'Keeffe
Paul J. O'Keeffe Pty Ltd, Brookvale, NSW Australia

1. Introduction

The Medpor Nasal Shell, available from Porex Surgical, Inc., now a Stryker company, was designed to reconstruct a saddle nose and produce an anatomically correct shape. The breakdown of the nasal shape that was used is illustrated in **Figure 1**. The shell does not extend into the tip in order to allow normal sideways movement of the tip.

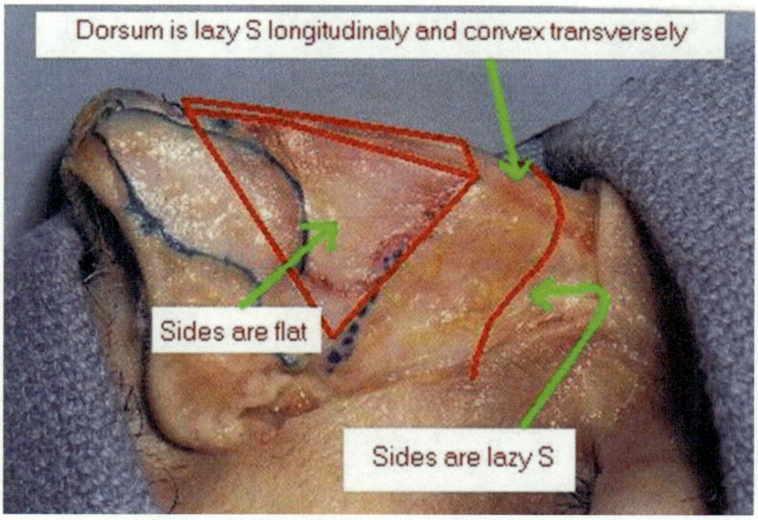

Fig. 1. Analysis of nasal shape for implant mould manufacture

The original version was first implanted in March 1999. It was thicker than the current thin shell as seen in **Figure 2** and it came with Medpor inserts that could be used to fill the void beneath the shell, **Figure 3**. Both thick and thin shells are provided with a blue silicone template **Figure 4** that can be inserted and then trimmed to a suitable dimension for the particular case. The silicone template is removed and placed over the actual implant for accurate trimming.

Eighty thick implants were placed between March 1999 and April 2005. The reconstructed noses were excellent aesthetically, **Figure 5**, and the nose tips were naturally flexible. Unfortunately, the movement between the reconstructed nasal pyramid and the nose tip resulted in implant exposure in 3 cases. The hard edge of the implant eroded through the underlying lining, **Figure 6**. Trimming the exposed Medpor initially corrected the problem but re-exposure and infection occurred months later. These infected implants were removed and the nasal pyramids were reconstructed with cartilage grafts.

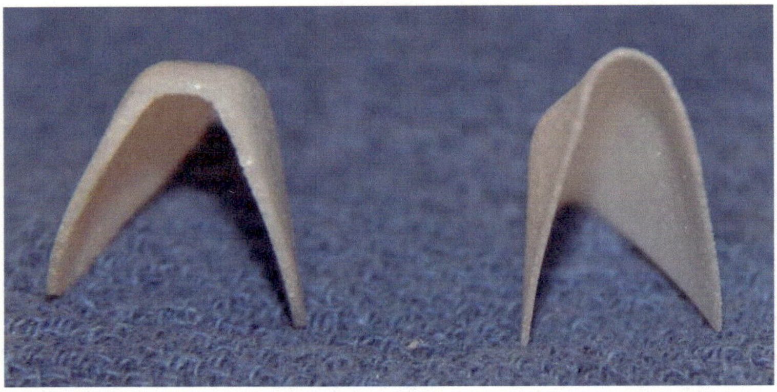

Fig. 2. Original thick Nasal Shell on left and new thin version on right

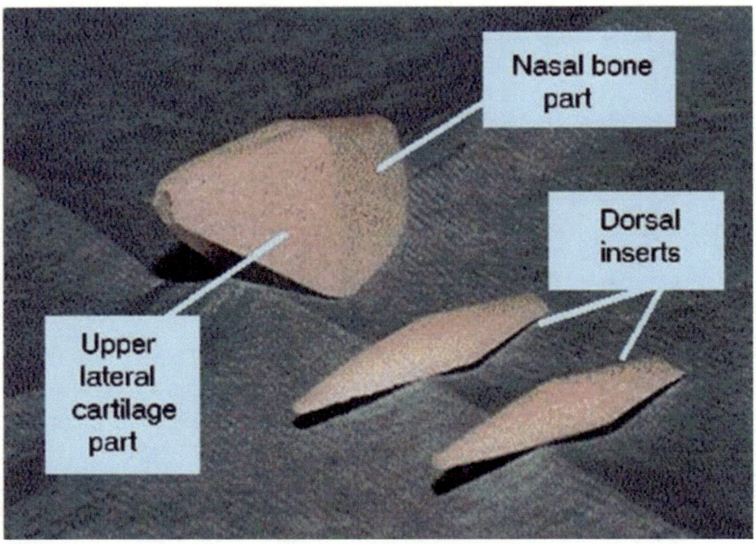

Fig. 3. Original Nasal Shell with inserts

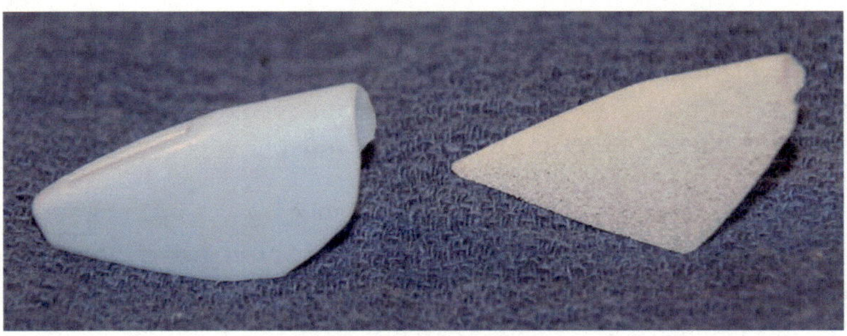

Fig. 4. Blue silicone template on left and thin shell on right

The thin Medpor Nasal Shell was designed to overcome the problems of the thicker and stiffer original Nasal Shell. The Medpor is universally thin allowing for a greater trimming of the implant, **Figure 7.** The implant is used now more as a cartilage graft forming device. Cartilage fragments are placed in the void beneath the thin shell and are expected to consolidate and grow to fill the void, **Figure 8**. If necessary, the Nasal Shell could then be removed leaving the patient with a perfectly shaped nasal pyramid. To date, very few implants have been removed but one was in response to recurrent sterile effusions. The shell was removed 13 months after implantation leaving a well formed nose **Figure 9**.

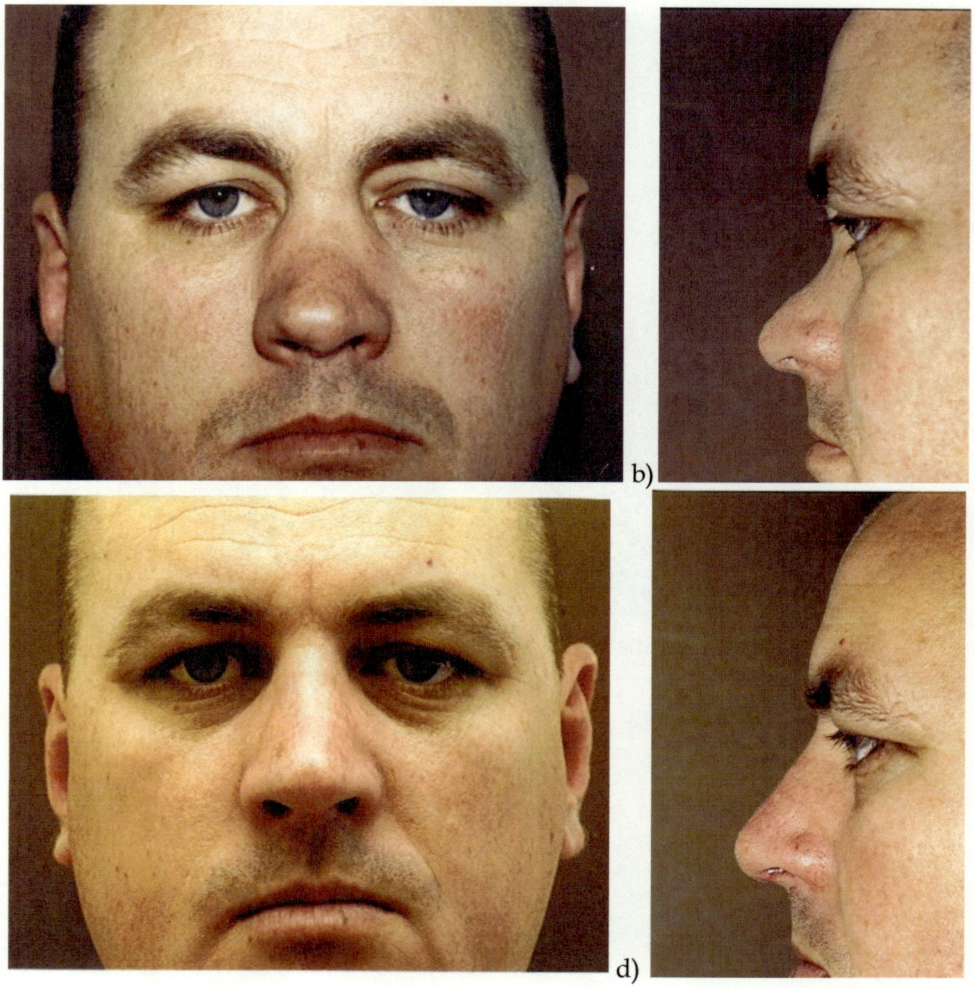

a) b) c) d)

Fig. 5. a and b show patient with a saddle nose, c and d show the post-operative result with the original Nasal Shell

The Thin Nasal Shell was first implanted in April 2004 and, since then, 98 have been placed. Every implant was trimmed, usually 25%, but sometimes more than this. The trimming is done mostly at the caudal end of the implant where a cartilage extender graft is attached, **Figure 10**. The implant composite is placed over the existing deformed nasal pyramid and then cartilage fragments are placed in the void.

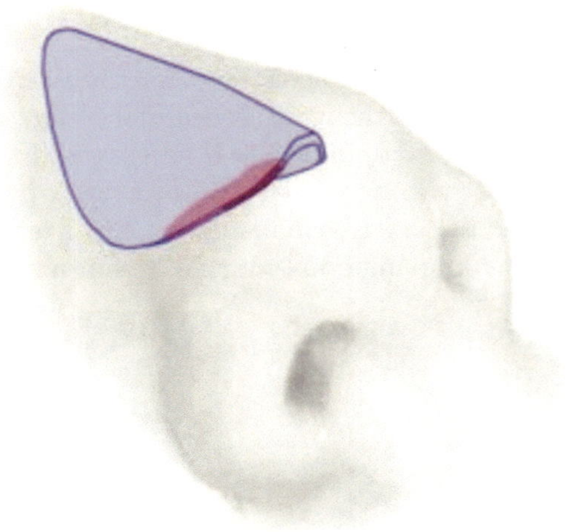

Fig. 6. Red area depicts exposed edge of Nasal Shell

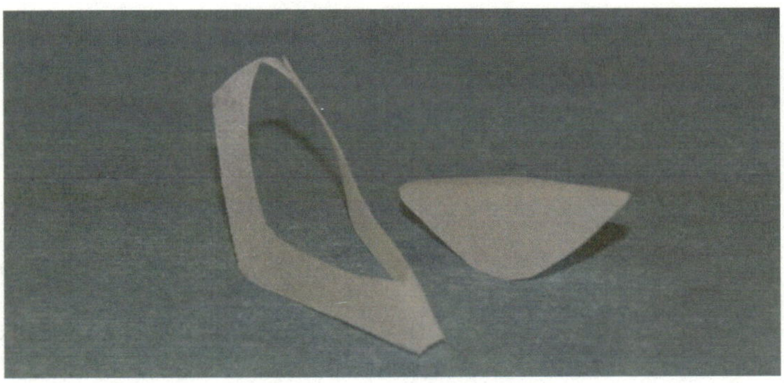

Fig. 7. A trimmed Thin Nasal Shell

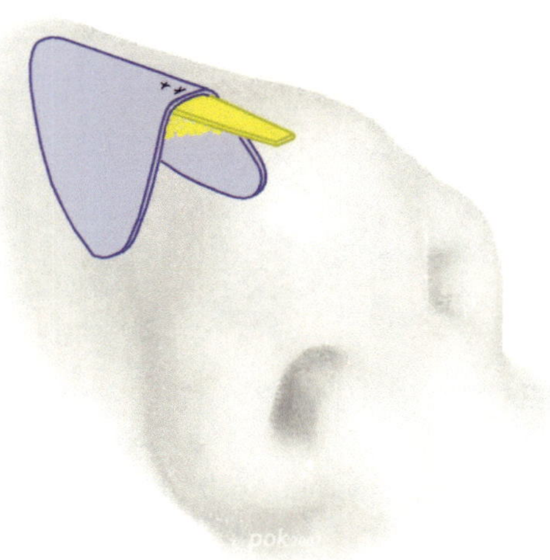

Fig. 8. A Thin Nasal Shell in situ with a cartilage extender graft and diced cartilage in the void

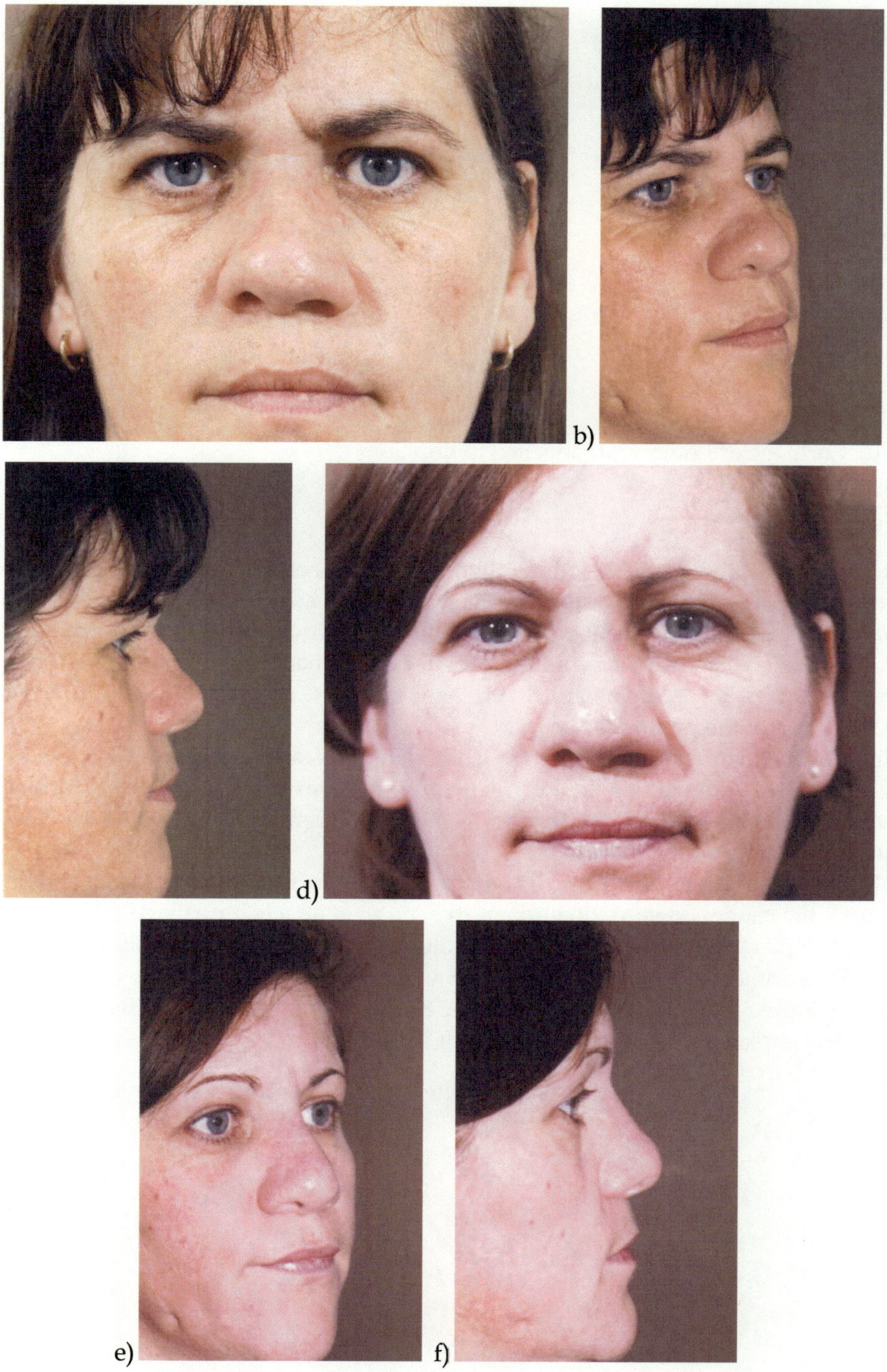

Fig. 9. a, b and c show a patient with a twisted costal cartilage graft in the nasal dorsum. d, e and f show post-operative result after removal of the implant. The cartilage graft associated with the implant has consolidated into a shape the patient is happy with

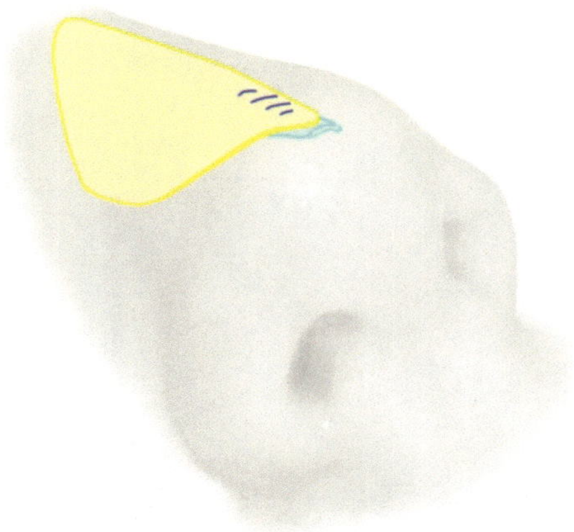

Fig. 10. Cartilage extender graft attached to implant

2. Technique

Nasal reconstruction with the Thin Medpor Nasal Shell plus cartilage graft is usually performed under general anaesthesia. The anaesthetist administers an intravenous dose of antibiotic at the commencement of the procedure, usually cephalothin sodium, 1g.

Cartilage is harvested from the septum, ears or ribs, in that order of preference. The nose tip is reconstructed by placement of cartilage graft as necessary before proceeding to reconstruction of the pyramid.

A blue silicone template comes with the Thin Medpor Nasal Shell, **Figure 4**. It can be placed over the nasal pyramid via intercartilaginous incisions. The template is trimmed to a suitable size for the nasal reconstruction. The template is then removed and used as a guide for trimming the Medpor implant.

The Medpor is trimmed in two stages, first to match the size of the template and second to trim back the caudal edge of the implant to expose an attached cartilage graft. The initially trimmed implant is soaked in antibiotic solution, 1g cephalothin sodium in 5ml normal saline. The cartilage graft is then sutured beneath the distal portion of the implant using 6-0 Prolene sutures. The implant is then further trimmed to leave the cartilage graft projecting beyond the implant edge as an extender graft, **Figure 11.**

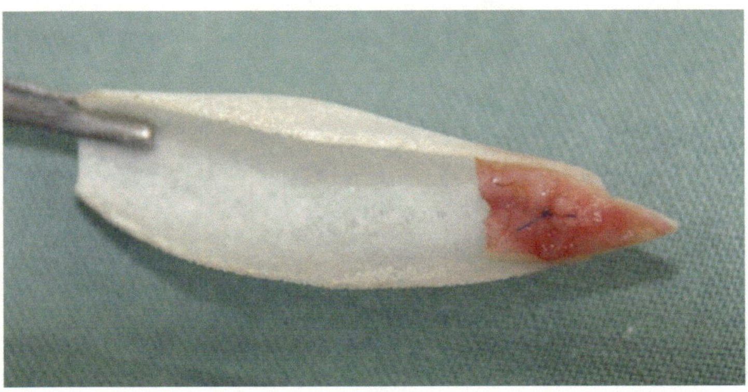

Fig. 11. Cartilage extender sutured to implant with 6/0 Prolene sutures

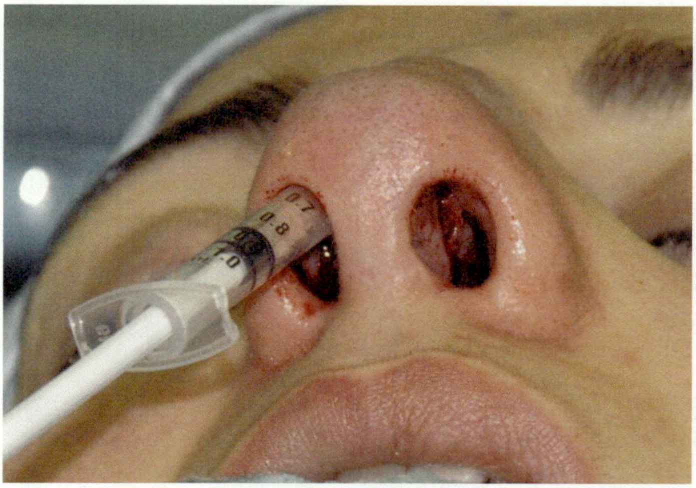

Fig. 12. Inserting diced cartilage into the void beneath the implant with a cut off 1ml syringe

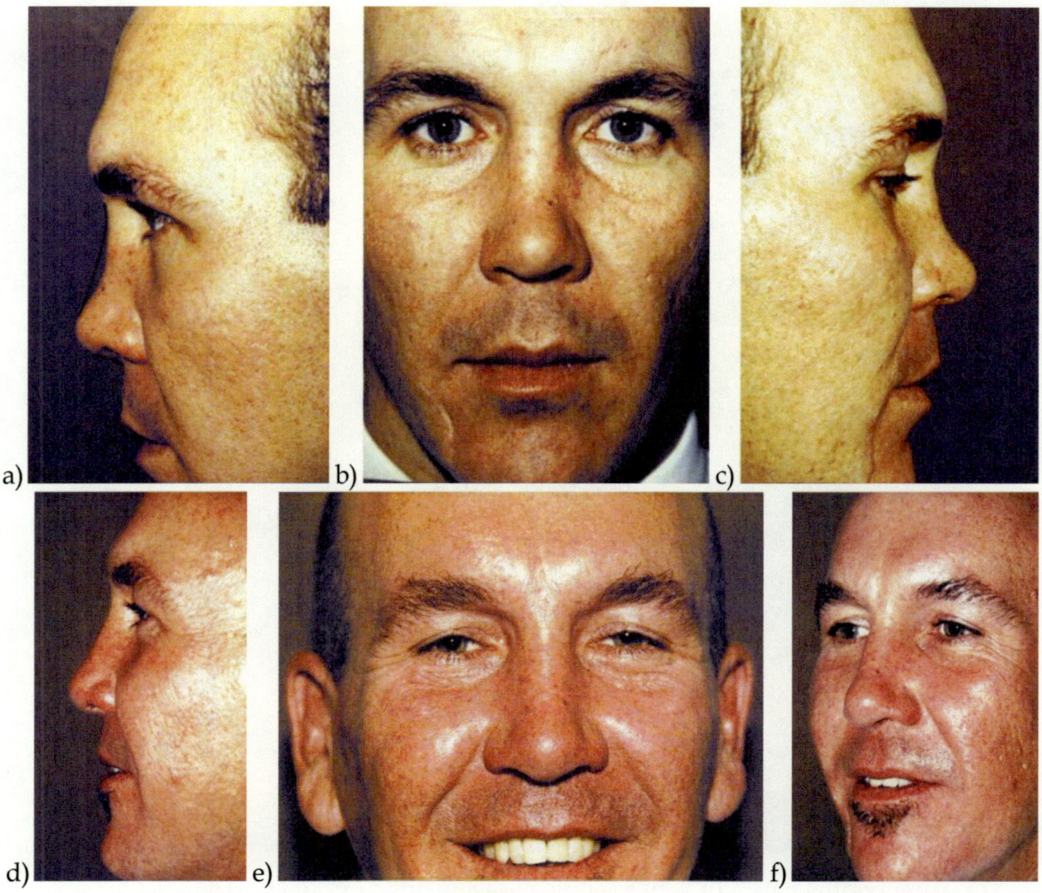

Fig. 13. a, b and c show a patient with a saddle nose. d, e and f show post-operative result following reconstruction with Thin Nasal Shell and cartilage grafts

The blue silicone template is reinserted into the nose and then partially extracted. The Nasal Shell and attached cartilage graft is then carefully inserted into the nose by sliding it over the template. The template is then removed.

Cartilage fragments are placed beneath the implant to partially fill the void. **Figure 12.** It is important to never overfill the void with cartilage fragments[1] as they act like ball bearings and the implant is likely to displace. The implant can be secured by suturing the cartilage extender graft to the nasal septum. Some of the antibiotic solution used for soaking the implant is drawn up and injected in the pocket over the implant.

Incisions are sutured with 4-0 plain catgut and a suitable nasal splint is applied. Post-operative antibiotics are given intravenously while an intravenous line is in place and then oral antibiotics are administered, usually Keflex 500mg three times a day for five days.

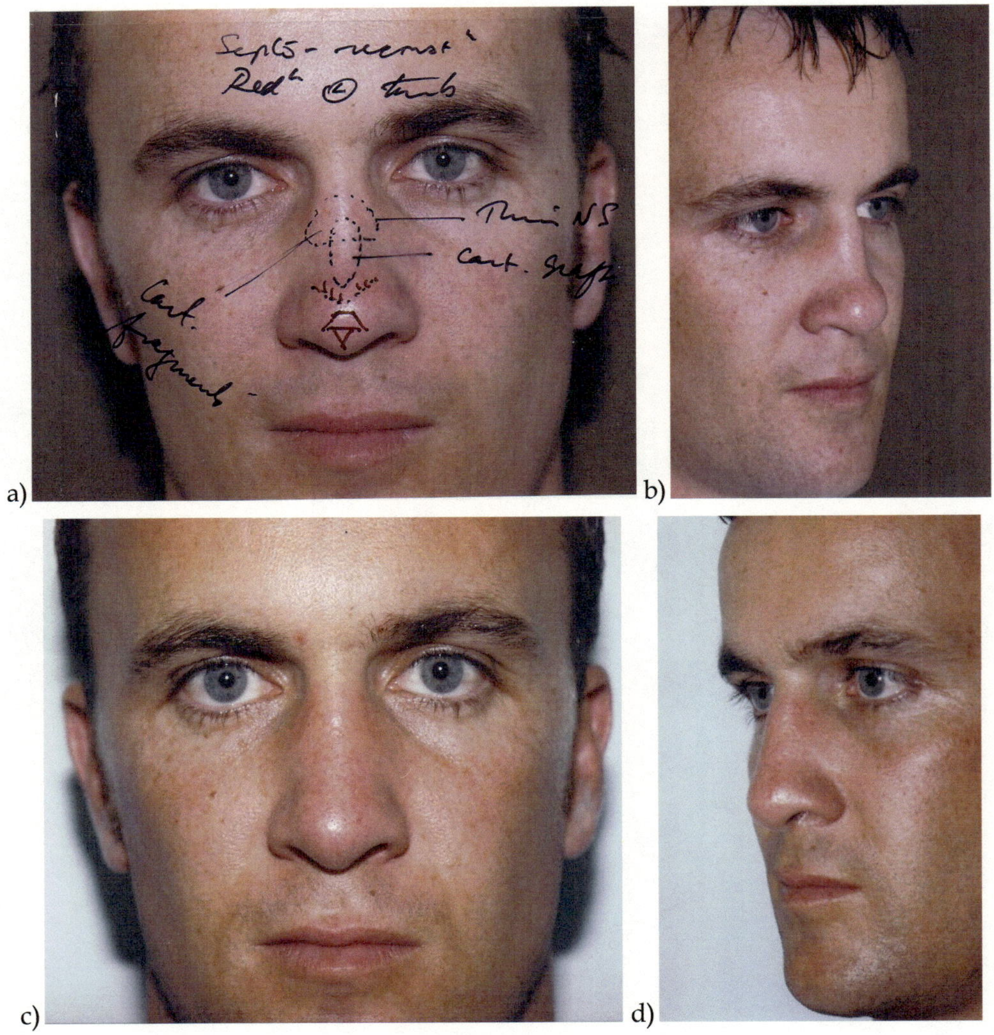

Fig. 14. a and b show a patient with a saddle nose and operative plan drawn on the photos. c and d show post-operative result following reconstruction with Thin Nasal Shell and cartilage grafts

3. Results

There have been no exposures or infections of the 98 Thin Medpor Nasal Shells. Some implants displaced presumably due to over packing cartilage fragments in the void beneath the implant. Those implants were repositioned. The remaining implants have been stable since restricting filling of the void to approximately 60% with fragmented cartilage.
One patient had recurrent sterile effusions, **Figure 9**. This implant was removed 13 months after placement and the effusions disappeared. The resultant nasal shape was excellent and has been maintained indicating consolidation of the graft beneath the implant.
Airways have been improved by placement of the Thin Medpor Nasal Shell. The implant acts as an umbrella and maintains patency of the nasal valves.

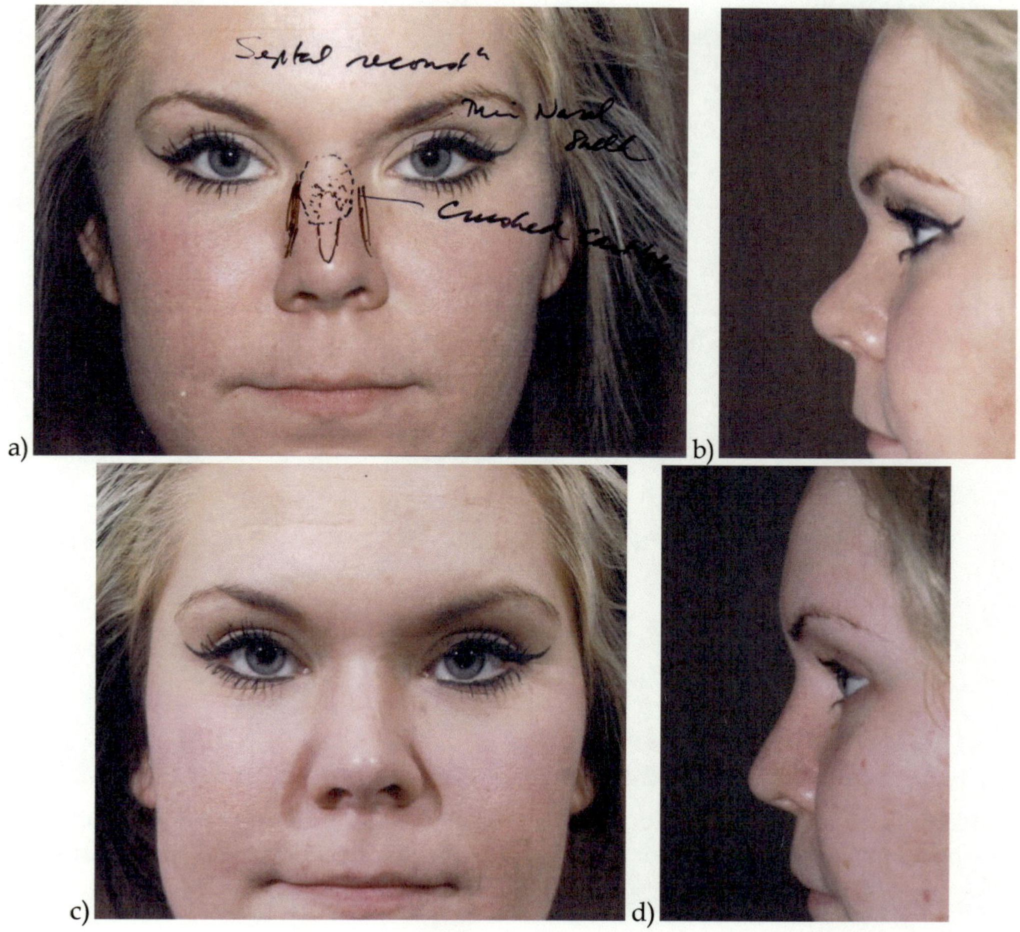

Fig. 15. a and b show a patient with a saddle nose. c and d show post-operative result following reconstruction with Thin Nasal Shell and cartilage grafts

Patients who had misgivings about placement of an implant in their nose were reassured that their implant could be removed after consolidation of the graft beneath it. None of these patients have come forth postoperatively to request removal of their implant. Should removal ever become necessary it is possible because the outer surface of the implant,

although perforated, is smooth. Separation from the overlying tissue is relatively easy. The under surface is rougher but separation from deep tissue is easy enough after outer surface separation because the shell is thin and very little tissue is entrapped into its structure.
A typical patient might have a saddle nose following trauma, **Figures 13a, 13b, 13c.** The patient is obviously happy with the postoperative result, **Figures 13d, 13e, 13f. Figures 14** to **16** show similarly satisfied patients. All have improved airways.

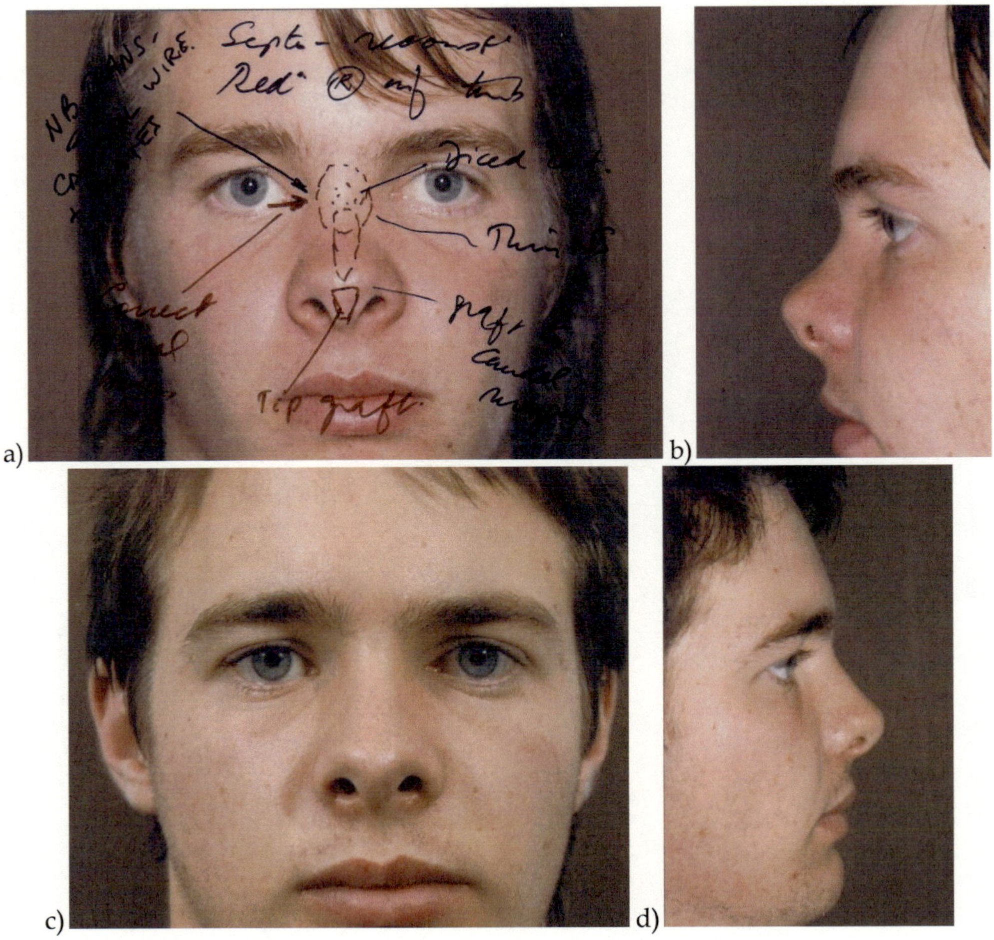

Fig. 16. a and b show a patient with a saddle nose and the detailed operative plan. c and d show post-operative result following reconstruction with Thin Nasal Shell and cartilage grafts

4. Discussion

A conventional approach to reconstruction of a saddle nose is to use the patient's own tissue with preference for septal cartilage before ear cartilage, ear cartilage before costal cartilage and costal cartilage before bone graft[2]. Bone graft is least preferred due to its tendency to atrophy over time[3,4,5,6]. Foreign implants have been shunned for nasal reconstruction by many surgeons in North America[7,8] but their use in Asia is more accepted[9,10]. An explanation for this difference is the likelihood of trauma being involved in the case of a Caucasian patient who has a saddle nose[11]. The scarred nasal tissue may allow easier ingress of bacteria into the pocket containing the implant and result in a relatively high post-operative infection rate. Bacteria in a pocket containing cartilage or bone graft are less likely to result in clinical infection[12,13].

Restricting the reconstruction options for a Caucasian patient may not always produce the best result. Available cartilage graft may not perfectly match the ideal shape of a nasal pyramid and bone grafts are often made too large cephalically and they are too hard caudally. It is preferable to reconstruct the nasal pyramid with an object that matches normal shape and which has bony consistency in its cephalic portion and cartilaginous consistency in its caudal portion[14]. The Thin Nasal Shell with a cartilage extender attached meets this need.

Previous nasal implants have been solid objects that rest on the nasal pyramid. Pressure atrophy of the underlying bone[15,16] can occur resulting in a flatter saddle nose than before should the implant be removed to treat infection. The Thin Nasal Shell overcomes this problem by being a shell under which cartilage fragments can be placed in order for them to consolidate into an ideal shape. The nose will be a better shape than before should it be necessary to remove this implant.

The Nasal Shell was specifically designed to reconstruct only the nasal pyramid, not the nose tip. The purpose was to simulate a natural nose and allow natural movement of the tip. This limits the possibility of changing the position of the tip but, of course, a long cartilage extender can be attached in order to push the tip caudally and lengthen a short nose. In any case, more cartilage will be available for grafting into the tip because less is used in the pyramid[17].

Familiarity with the Nasal Shell advances its position on the surgeon's preference list of reconstruction options. Initially the shell will be on the bottom of the list but after rewarding results are seen it will move up the list. The author places the thin Nasal Shell plus cartilage graft after septal or auricular cartilage alone. It is far superior to bone grafts in the author's experience over 40 years.

The elegance of results makes the shell suitable for patients with thin skin. Poorly shaped bone or cartilage grafts can be obvious unless masked with dermis or fascia grafts[18,19]. It is rarely necessary to place such masking grafts over a nasal shell.

5. Conclusion

The Thin Medpor Nasal Shell used in conjunction with cartilage grafts is an excellent means for reconstruction of the nasal pyramid. The resultant nasal shape is anatomical and the umbrella effect of the implant ensures an unobstructed airway. Less donor cartilage is needed for nasal pyramid reconstruction thereby reducing donor site morbidity and leaving more cartilage graft for associated tip reconstruction.

6. References

[1] Erol, Ö. Onur. The Turkish Delight: A Pliable Graft for Rhinoplasty Plastic & Reconstructive Surgery. 105(6):2229-2241, May 2000.

[2] Sajjadian, Ali; Rubinstein, Roee; Naghshineh, Nima. Current Status of Grafts and Implants in Rhinoplasty: Part I. Autologous Grafts Plastic & Reconstructive Surgery. 125(2):40e-49e, February 2010

[3] Phillips, J. H., and Rahn, B. A. Fixation effects on membranous and endochondral onlay bone-graft resorption. Plast. Reconstr. Surg. 82: 872, 1988.
[4] Holmström, Hans; Gewalli, Fredrik. Long-Term Behavior of Three Different Grafts in Nasomaxillary Reconstruction of Binder Syndrome: An Analysis by Digitalized Measurements Plastic & Reconstructive Surgery. 122(5):1524-1534, November 2008.
[5] Farina, R., and Villano, J. B. Follow-up of bone grafts to the nose. Plast. Reconstr. Surg. 48: 251, 1971
[6] Rune, B., and Aberg, M. Bone grafts to the nose in Binder's syndrome (maxillonasal dysplasia): A follow-up of eleven patients with the use of profile roentgenograms. Plast. Reconstr. Surg. 101: 297, 1998
[7] Ziv M. Peled, Anne G. Warren, Patrick Johnston, Michael J. Yaremchuk. The Use of Alloplastic Materials in Rhinoplasty Surgery: A Meta-Analysis. Plast. Reconstr. Surg. 121: 85e, 2008.
[8] Daniel, R. K. The role of diced cartilage grafts in rhinoplasty. Aesthetic Surg. J. 26: 209, 2006
[9] Deva, A. K., Merten, S., and Chang, L. Silicone in nasal augmentation rhinoplasty: A decade of clinical experience. Plast. Reconstr. Surg. 102: 1230, 1998.
[10] Lam, S. M., and Kim, Y. K. Augmentation rhinoplasty of the Asian nose with the "bird" silicone implant. Ann. Plast. Surg. 51: 249, 2003.
[11] Herbst, Andrew. Extrusion of An Expanded Polytetrafluoroethylene Implant After Rhinoplasty Plastic & Reconstructive Surgery. 104(1):295-296, July 1999.
[12] Maas CS, Monhian N, Shah SB. Implants in rhinoplasty. Facial Plast Surg. 1997;13:279–290.
[13] Sajjadian, Ali; Naghshineh, Nima; Rubinstein, Roee. Current Status of Grafts and Implants in Rhinoplasty: Part II. Homologous Grafts and Allogenic Implants Plastic & Reconstructive Surgery. 125(3):99e-109e, March 2010.
[14] Daniel, R. K. Rhinoplasty and rib grafts: Evolving a flexible operative technique. Plast. Reconstr. Surg. 94: 597-609, 1994
[15] Yanagisawa, Akihiro; Nakamura, Toshitaka; Arakaki, Minoru; Yano, Hiroki; Yamashita, Shunichi; Fujii, Tohru. Migration of Hydroxyapatite Onlays into the Mandible and Nasal Bone and Local Bone Turnover in Growing Rabbits Plastic & Reconstructive Surgery. 99(7):1972-1982, June 1997.
[16] Matarasso, Alan; Elias, Arthur C.; Elias, Richard L. Labial Incompetence: A Marker for Progressive Bone Resorption in Silastic Chin Augmentation: An Update Plastic & Reconstructive Surgery. 112(2):676-678, August 2003.
[17] Hodgkinson, Darryl J. Cranial Bone Grafts for Dorsal Nasal Augmentation Plastic & Reconstructive Surgery. 104(5):1570, October 1999.
[18] Miller, Timothy A Temporalis Fascia Grafts for Facial and Nasal Contour Augmentation. Plastic & Reconstructive Surgery. 81(4):524-533, April 1988.
[19] Guerrerosantos, J. Temporoparietal free fascia grafts in rhinoplasty. Plast. Reconstr. Surg. 74: 465, 1984.

7

Surgical Management of Nasal Hemangiomas

Aleksandar Vlahovic
Plastic, Aesthetic and Reconstructive Surgery, Belgrade
Serbia

1. Introduction

Vascular anomalies are seen in all branches of medicine and surgery. The term vascular anomaly is necessarily broad, encompassing lesions of skin and viscera and excluding abnormalities of the heart and large arteries and veins [1]. A biologic classification of vascular anomalies described in 1982 by Mulliken and Glovacki, correlates the cellular features of vascular anomalies with clinical characteristics and natural history [1,2]. Vascular anomalies of infancy and childhood are divided into two major categories: 1) tumors (most being hemangiomas) and 2) vascular malformations [1].

The typical infantile hemangiomas (IHs) appears postnataly and evolve through 3 predictable stages: a rapidly proliferating stage (generally lasting 8 to 12 months), followed by prolonged involuting phase (1 to 7 years), entering the involuted phase characterized by fibrofatty residuum [1,3]. Early proliferative-stage hemangiomas are composed of well-defined, but noncapsulated, masses of plump endothelial cells and attendant pericytes that form small lumina containing erythrocytes. Even in early lesional stage, endothelium posses immunophenotypic and ultrastructural features of mature endothelium including immunoreactivity for CD31, CD 34, factor VIII- related antigen *Ulex europeaus* lectin I, VE-cadherin, HLA-DR, and vimentin. GLUT 1 is specific and useful immunohistochemical marker for hemangiomas during all phases of these lesions [3]. The typical IHs appears postnatally, grows rapidly, and regresses slowly. The term congenital hemangioma was introduced to denote a vascular tumor that had grown to its maximum size at birth and does not exhibit accelerated postnatal growth. There are at least two major subgroups: rapidly involuting congenital hemangioma (RICH), and noninvoluting congenital hemangioma (NICH) [4].

Infantile hemangiomas (IHs), are the most common benign, soft tissue tumors of infancy which affect between 4 and 12% of all Caucasian [1,5,6]. The prevalence among Asians and black infants is considerably less [5]. There is a 3:1 predilection for the female sex, and they are weakly associated with prematurity [6–8]. The pathophysiologic mechanisms leading to endothelial cells proliferation and involution are poorly understood [6,7]. Current theories focus on progenitor cells, development field defects, placental involvement, derangement of angiogenesis and mutations in the cytokine regulatory pathway [6,7]. Involution coincides with increased apoptosis of endothelial and stromal cells [7].

Most IHs involve the head and neck (up to 60%) [1]. Facial IHs are associated with parental reactions of disbelief and fear, particularly in the growth phase. Most parents expressed a desire to have the hemangioma removed before the children entered school. The strangers often raised the question of child abuse, and some parents indicated that their children try to hide their lesions from the other [8].

Clinical appearance allows differentiation between focal, indeterminate and segmental IHs. Size, location and subtype were major factors that predicted complications and need for treatment [9]. Focal type had a tumor-like appearance and a less common diffuse type had a segmental distribution pattern and plaquelike appearance. Segmental IHs exhibit worse prognosis with more complications (ulceration, airway obstruction) [5,9]. Although subglottic hemangiomas are rare, they are extremely dangerous due to their location and rapid growth during the proliferative phase. "Beard" distribution of hemangioma is highly suspected for subglottic localization of hemangioma [5,6,23].

Most IHs are small, harmless tumors that should be allowed to involute without treatment. Generally, treatment is instituted for complications within the IHs itself (such as ulceration, bleeding, infection), or impairments caused by the hemangioma (amblyopia, impaired breathing, feeding difficulties, heart failure), and the wait-and-see medical management policy for these hemangioma should be replaced by a more active approach. [9,10]. More than half of IHs will involute with a poor result and therefore required a corrective surgery [11]. Haggstrom et al. stated that 43% patients with a facial hemangioma received treatment of some kind [9].

The management of hemangioma is an area of great controversy [6]. Current options are conservative treatment (corticosteroids, interferons, hemiotherapy, propranolol), laser treatment, and surgical treatment [6,9–27]. Corticosteroids were generally accepted to be the first-line therapy for hemangiomas [6]. They can be used orally, intralesionally, intravenously or topically. Interferons were usually reserved for serious cases in which steroids were contraindicated, have failed, or in severe complications [12]. Unfortunately, severe neurotoxicity (spastic diplegia) was found to be severe adverse effect [6]. Antineoplastic agents were also successful in treatment of hemangioma, because of their proliferative nature (bleomycin, cyclophosphamide, vinristine) but this treatment should be reserved for infants with hemangioma demonstrating aggressive behavior characteristics [6]. A wide variety of lasers have been used with a broad range of results (pulse-dye, CO2). Externally-applied laser can penetrate only 1-2 mm into the dermis and therefore has a limited value for the treatment of hemangioma [1,6]. Embolisation, cryotherapy and compression had also been used [6,12,16,30].

Recently propranolol proved itself effective in inducing regression of growing hemangioma. There are several reports confirming prompt response of hemangioma to propranolol with no major side effects [23,25,28,29].

There are three questions regarding surgical intervention: 1) what are the indications, 2) when it should be done (timing) and 3) how it should be done [30]. Surgical excision of hemangioma has been usually performed by lenticular excision with a linear closure. This technique is useful in the eyelid, lip and neck region [30]. An alternative technique that does not have these disadvantages is the circular excision or by circular excision and with purse string closure which is now considered the first line technique at any stage of the tumors life cycle [11,30].

In some children with extremely large hemangiomas, the vascularity of the lesion is also a significant anesthetic consideration. There is a need for particular attention to hemodynamic consideration with anesthesia and potential need for transfusion. Haemostatic squeezing suture around the hemangioma can be used prior to resection to avoid blood loss [23].

2. Nasal hemangiomas

Nasal hemangiomas are among the more distressing, if large, can cause a significant residual damage to the shape of the nose [6]. Due to their location, nasal hemangiomas are profoundly disturbing lesions both for patients and their families (Fig. 1). Hemangiomas involving the nose occur approximately 15,8% of facial hemangiomas [13]. The nasal tip is by far the most common site of nasal hemangiomas [11].

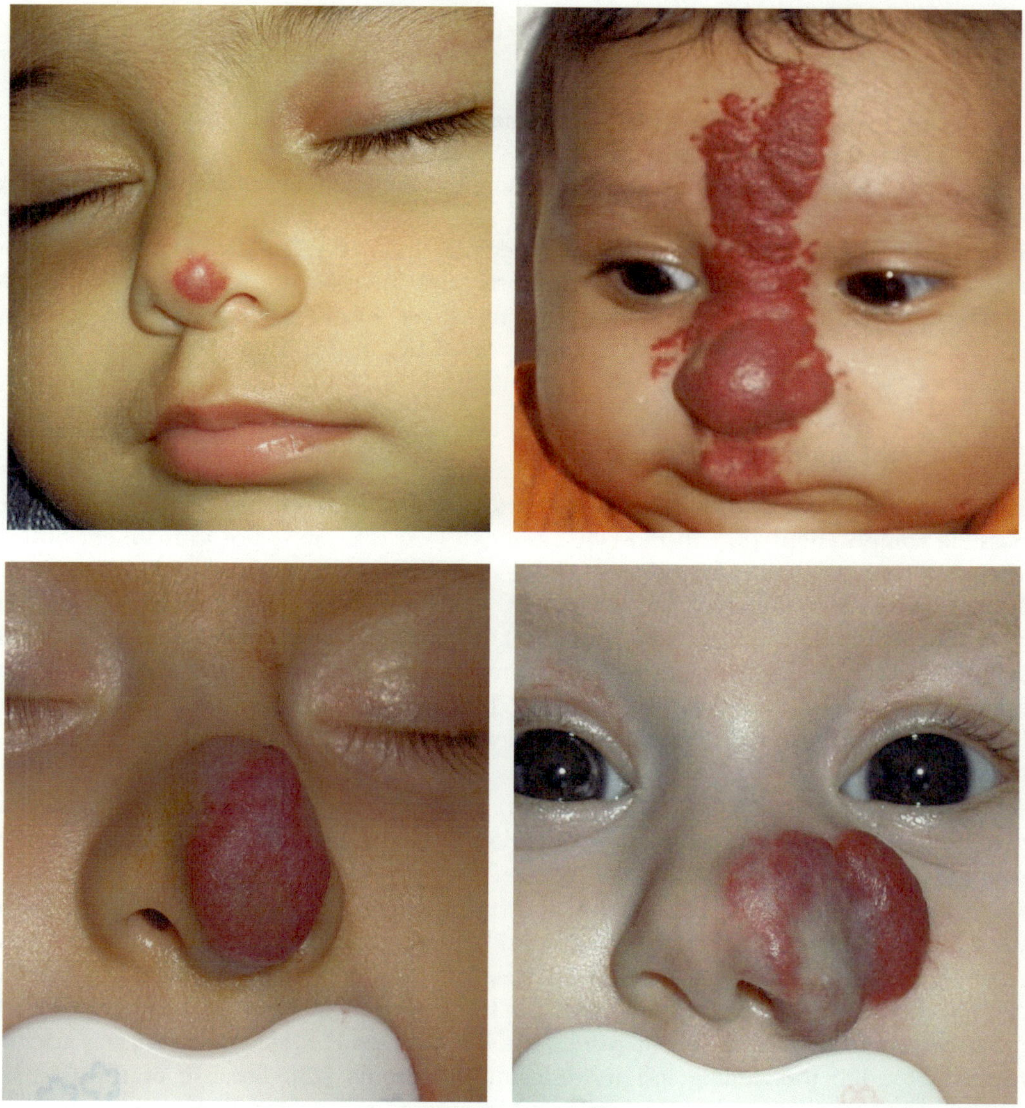

Fig. 1. Different types of nasal hemangioma from small no harming, involving nasal tip, complicated with nasal obstruction and large superficial hemangioma

Nasal hemangiomas can cause functional problems (nasal obstruction, alteration of the nasal valve, ulceration and destruction of the delicate growing cartilage of the nose) and severe psychological sequelae to the children because of social redicule of their peers, and also from medical professionals who are using terms like "Cyrano nose, "Pinocchio nose". During proliferative phase they can permanently distort nasal architecture (by displacing lower lateral cartilages laterally) [13-15,17]. Parent's anxiety is something that surgeon have to deal with during the child growth. In most cases they are not satisfied with explanation that hemangioma will regress spontaneously during childhood. Aesthetic problem is usually obvious. Eivazi et al. classified nasal tip hemangiomas as „limited" or „advanced" [25]. Hamou et al. identify three types of nasal hemangiomas that lead to three distinct surgical approaches:

- Type A (mild cases): no cutaneous involvement, no misalignment of the cartilages an mild nasal volume increase
- Type B (moderate cases): partial cutaneous infiltration, misalignment of the cartilages and moderate nasal volume increase
- Type C (severe cases): cutaneous infiltration, misalignment of the cartilages and severe nasal volume increase [31].

They are usually subcutaneous or mixed superficial and subcutaneous lesions that occupy the space between the skin and the nasal tip and lower lateral cartilages [15]. Nasal hemangioma are often slow to regress, leaving excess wrinkled nonelastic skin, residual fibrofatty tissue with a permanently bulbous nasal tip, visible teleangiectases or contour deficiencies [11,13,14,17,19,20,27].

3. Treatment options

The treatment of nasal hemangiomas is extremely difficult because of its location and possible complications [31]. In most of these cases expectation is not a treatment option. There is a pressure from the family to improve the child's appearance.

Numerous medical and surgical treatment approaches have been proposed for the treatment of these tumors. The treatment choices of nasal hemangiomas are still controversial considering use of preoperative medical treatment, timing of surgery, surgical approach and necessity of skin resection [15, 27].

Pharmacological, surgical or laser interventions are current treatment options for nasal hemangiomas [13-27].

A „no-touch" or conservative approach for the treatment of nasal hemangiomas was previously advocated with frequent consultations with the parents to furnish psychological support [26].

Advocates of conservative treatment claim that resection causes growth disturbances in nasal architecture [14,16]. Denk et al. consider that conservative treatment should be reserved for small hemangiomas on the nose that are not deforming and are without complications [17]. Corticosteroids were, for the long period, the first line treatment for nasal hemangioma with excellent results in 30% of cases [13,18]. Interferon was usually reserved for life threatening lesions resistant to steroids [13]. Because of the possible complications (skin atrophy) Hochman and Mascareno have moved away from using local steroid injections for nasal hemangioma [22].

Because of convincing results, beta blockers are preferred as the first treatment option for proliferating hemangioma [25,28,29,31]. Proponents of early surgery suggest that aesthetic and functional improvement during a critical period in child development can be achieved [13-17].

Laser is indicated only for the treatment of the involuting hemangioma, and it is not helpful for the deeper components [12,16].

4. Surgical treatment

Thomson et al. have been treated eleven patients with different surgical approaches. Several procedures had been carried out on each patient (an average of 4 operations on one patient) with 50% delayed primary healing, especially in earlier operated patients [26].

Van der Meulen et al. moved away from „no touch" approach, and they stated „that there is no need to wait with effective treatment until involution has stopped". They had 9 patients operated with low-flying bird incision (Rethi incision), and with so called „L-approach", which is Rethi incision extended in cranial direction along the alar fold and nasomaxillary junction. They performed before school age without previous conservative treatment [19].

Pitanguy advocated an elliptical midline incision over the dorsum of the nose that can give good functional results but with obvious midline scar on the back of the nose, and the excision of the dog ear may cause extensions of the incision up into the glabellar region, which may lead to an unsatisfactory aesthetic result [20,24].

Jackson presented excision of a nasal tip hemangioma via open rhinoplasty procedure, with step incision on columella, proceeding on both sides of columella, and continuing just inside the alar rims. The resection of hemangioma and fibrofatty tissue begins between the medial crura and continues upwards over the domes of lower lateral cartilages. The medial crura and the domes of the lower lateral cartilages are approximated with nonapsorbable suture. Intranasal incisions are closed with absorbable suture. A plaster cast was placed for seven days. Care must be taken not to remove too much tissue because with the time and continued involution, this may lead to loss of the nasal projection. The excess skin is allowed to contract over the time (six months) [24].

Denk et al. used the incision made in midline, staring at the tip of the nose, extending the incision superiorly or inferiorly as needed. The mean age at the first operation was 2,2 years [17].

Warren et al. stated that the nose may be divided into topographic subunits (dorsum, tip, alar lobules, side-walls, and soft triangles). There incision were placed along the the lines that separate this subunits. The incision placement in this modified subunit approach to nasal tip hemangiomas was at lateral aspect of the nasal dorsum and carried down around the tip in the declivity medial to the alar lobule and medially into the infratip intercrucial region [15].

Faguer et al. suggest for surgical treatment of nasal hemangiomas transcolumellar low-flying bird (Rethi incision), combined with rim incision to expose alar cartilages [21]. With this technique they manage to excise small and large hemangiomas. Waner at al. stated that this approach is less appropriate for larger hemangioma, because the the incision cannot be extended cranially [13].

McCarthy et al. performed surgical resection of nasal tip hemangioma when the patients was over the age of 3 years for the treatment of lesions that showed no signs of regression over at least a 6 month period. „Open rhinoplasty approach" was used similar to Faguer et al. with transcolumellar incision and marginal „rim incision". Before this haemostatic sutures around the lesion were placed. If there was marked skin excess after redraping, it was resected, sometimes with central wedge excision [14].

Waner et al. proposed modified subunit approach along the contour lines of nasal subunits. Their surgical approach is based on the principles of Burgett and Menick subunit surgery in reconstructive surgery of the nose, but the incision line has been modified to allow better access to all of nasal subunits, and to allow trimming of the excess skin after the hemangioma has been removed. By this technique the lower lateral cartilages are approximated, as well as the medial crura, narrowing the columella to achieve nasal projection. These author avoid placement of in incision in an anterior location due to aesthetic reasons, preserving if it is possible some part of the affected skin which can be treated by laser [13].

Hochman and Mascareno proposed the combination of several treatment modalities. They use classical surgical approach based on already accepted rules, extending the incisions into the alar grooves or vertically along junction of the nasal tip and lobular subunits or even up the midline of the tip [22].

Vlahovic and coworkers use the open rhinoplasty incision for nasal tip, columella and alar subunits hemangioma and circular excision and „purse string suture" for large nasal hemangioma localized on the nasal dorsum with predominant deep component with previous medical (corticosteroid) treatment for large hemangiomas [23].

Eivazi et al. suggested that propranolol should be used as a treatment option for hemangioma of the nasal tip, and if there is indication for surgical treatment (destructive, highly proliferative or otherwise uncontrollable lesions) it should be conventional and made on the basis of the affected regions [25].

Arneja et al. advocate combined medical and surgical approach to treat the „Cyrano" nose. An open rhinoplasty approach with skin resection is the authors preferred technique [27].

Hamou et al. advocate early surgery and the operative technique was chosen based on the size of the lesion and the presence or absence of cutaneous infiltration. [31].

5. Conclusion

The optimal treatment approach for nasal hemangiomas remains controversial. Management of nasal hemangiomas involves a combination of serial observation, conservative treatment (propranolol), and surgical therapy.

Serial observation is indicated for small nasal hemangioma, which requires no treatment, but in that way we can give support and counseling to the patient and family. As the results after treatment of hemangioma with propranolol are encouraging, the beta blockers are preferred as the first treatment option for proliferating IHs, and this includes nasal hemangiomas also.

In a rapidly growing hemangioma (precisely the hemangiomas that one would prefer not to operate upon due to increased vascularity and blood loss), the straightforward decision should be to give a trial with propranolol, before embarking upon surgery. If propranolol fails, then surgery becomes next option.

The treatment protocol for propranolol developed by Siegfried at al. to optimize the safety is as follows: baseline echocardiography and 48-hour hospitalization or home nursing visits to monitor vital signs and blood glucose levels, medication is given every 8 hours, with a initial dose of 0,16 mg per kilogram of body weight. If the vital signs and glucose levels remain normal, the dose is incrementally doubled to maximum of 0,67 mg per kilogram (to a maximum daily dose of 2.0 mg per kilogram). This therapy should be continued through the proliferative phase of haemangioma growth or until no further improvement occurs. Instead of abrupt discontinuation a gradual tapering of propranolol over 2-3 weeks is recommended. If a rebound effect occurs patients are placed back on propranolol [29].

Different surgical procedures have been suggested for the treatment of nasal hemangiomas depending on the size and location of hemangioma (Fig.2). Surgery had to be performed

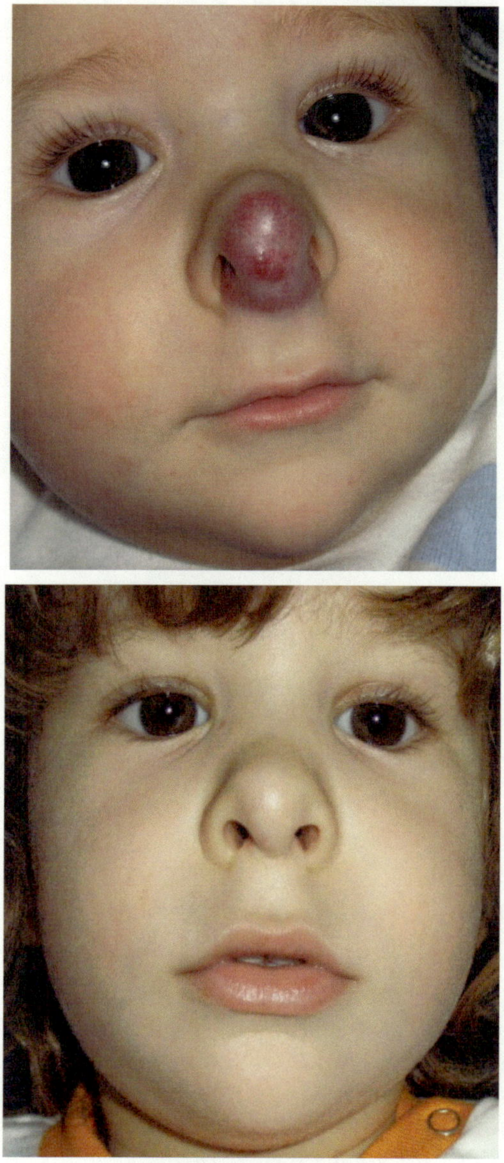

Fig. 2. Preoperative nasal hemangioma and result two years after open rhinotomy excision

under general anesthesia, with local infiltration of 1:100,000 adrenalin at the incision place. The selection of the optimal surgical approach should be made carefully on the basis of the affected regions. An open rhinoplasty approach, with or without skin resection, should be preferred technique for the lesion that involved nasal tip, columella and alar subunits, and in if wider approach is needed the nasal subunits had to be respected (Fig.3).

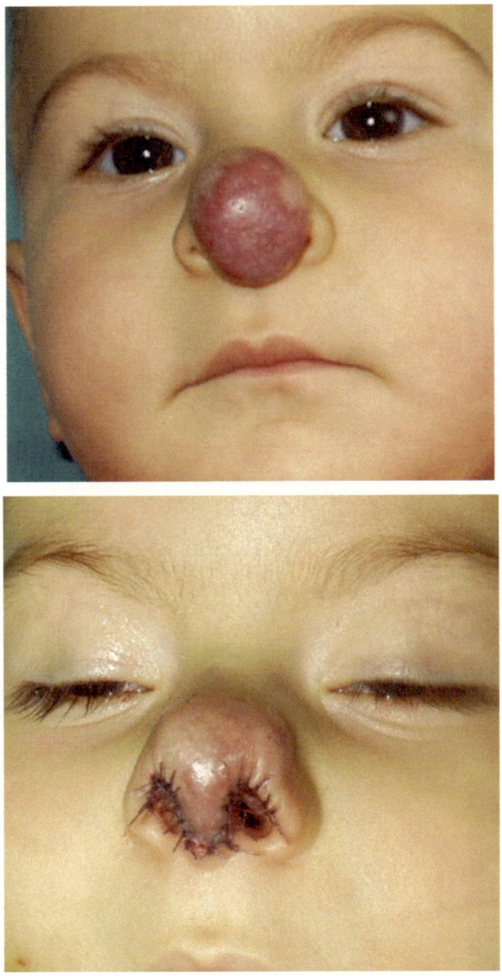

Fig. 3. Intraoperativne result after excision of nasal hemangioma with open rhinoplasty approach

Considering the timing of the surgery, early surgery at the end of the proliferative phase and during second year of life with maximum preservation of the tissue is appropriate because psychosocial, aesthetic and functional problems can be avoided. Surgical removal of nasal hemangioma should be delayed until the hemangioma has stopped proliferating. Surgical treatment during involutional phase is technically easier.

If there are no possibilities for total excision of hemangioma it can be reduced to an acceptable level avoiding destruction of the nasal tissue.

Subtotal excision for large hemangioma, without all of the affected skin, which will fade in the involutive phase, avoiding visible scars, by placing the incision along the columellar edge and parallel to the nostril is appropriate approach (Fig.4).

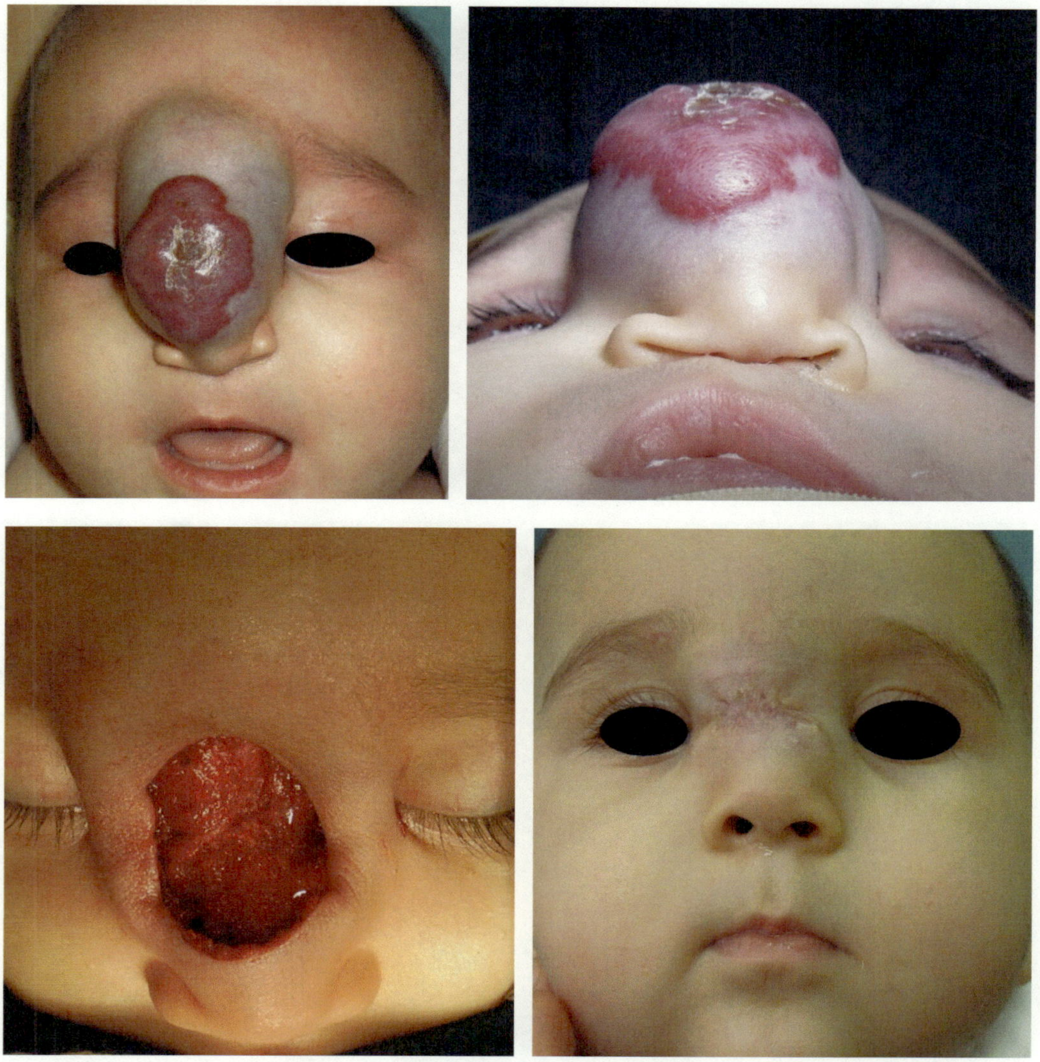

Fig. 4. Circular excision and „purse string suture" technique for large nasal hemangioma

If deep component of hemangioma is predominant, and hemangioma is mostly placed on the nasal dorsum, a circular excision and „purse string suture" technique will be appropriate because of „tissue expander" effect of hemangioma (Fig.5). The scar by this technique is more acceptable comparing to lenticular excision especially for large hemangiomas.
Surgery will retain its importance in cases of non responders to beta blockers, or the theoretical remaining deformity caused by the residual hemangioma or remnant fibrous fatty tissue after hemangiomas regression.

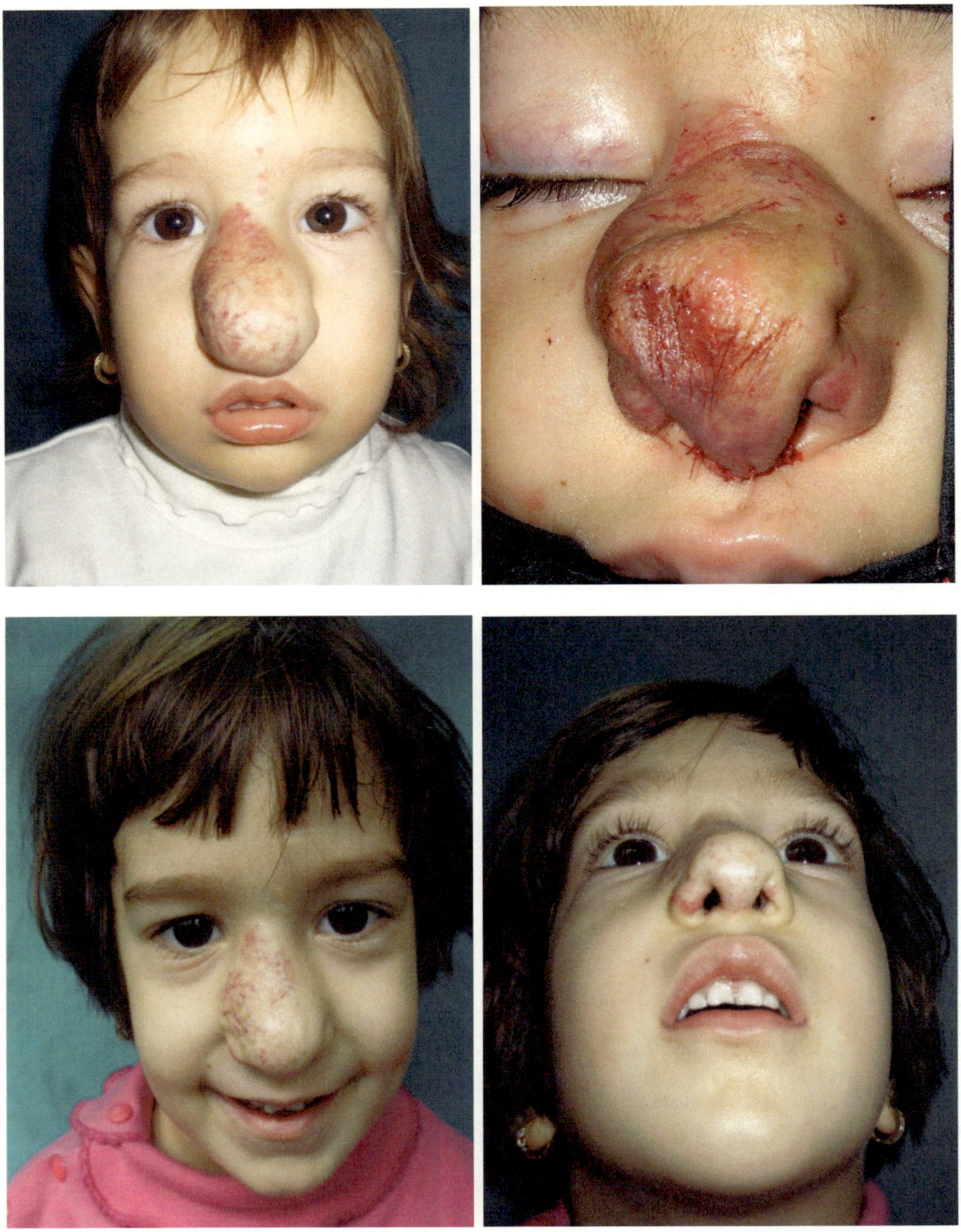

Fig. 5. Excision of large nasal hemangioma with open rhinoplasty approach, minimal tissue removing, result after two years

6. References

[1] SJ Fishman, JB Mulliken. Vascular anomalies. Ped Clin N Am 1998;45(6):1455-1477.

[2] JB Mlliken, J Glowacki. Hemangiomas and vascular malfomations in infants and children:a classification based on endothelial characteristics. Plast Reconstr Surg 1982; 69(3):412-422.
[3] PE North, M Waner, A Mizeracki, MC Mihm. GLUT 1:a newly discovered immunohistochemical marker for juvenile hemangiomas. Hum Pathol 2000;31(1):11-22.
[4] JB Mulliken, O Enjolras. Congenital hemangiomas and infantile hemangioma:missing links. J Am Acad Dermatol 2004;50(6):875-882.
[5] M Waner, PE North, KA Scherer, IJ Frieden, A Waner MC Mihm Jr.The nonrandom distribution of facial hemangimas. Arch Dermatol 2003;139:869-875.
[6] AL Bruckner, IJ Frieden. Infantile hemangiomas. J A Acad Dermatol 2006; 55(4):671-682.
[7] CG Bauland, MA. van Steensel, PM Steijlen, PNMA Rieu, PHM Spauwen. The pathogenesis of hemangiomas:review. Plast Reconstr Surg 2006;117(2):29-35.
[8] JL Tanner, MP Dechert, IJ Frieden. Growing up with a facial hemangioma: parent and child coping and adaptation. Pediatr 1998; 101(3):446-52.
[9] AN Haggstrom, BA Drolet, E Baselga, SL Chamlin, MC Garzon, KA Horii, AW Lucky, AJ Mancini, DW Metry, B Newell AJ Nopper, IJ Frieden. Prospective study of infantile hemangiomas: Clinical characteristics predicting complications and treatment. Pediatr 2006;118(3):882-87.
[10] CG Bauland, JM Smit, R Ketelaars, PNMA Rieu, PHM Spauwen. Management of hemangiomas of infancy: a retrospective analysis and treatment protocol. Scand. J Plast Reconstr Surg Hand Surg. 2008;42:86-91.
[11] M Waner, L Buckmiller, JY Suen. Surgical management of hemangiomas of the head and neck. Oper Tech Otolar-Head Neck Surg 2002;13(1):77-84.
[12] A Vlahovic, R Simic, Dj Kravljanac. Circular excision and purse string suture technique in the management of facial hemangiomas. Int J Ped Otolar 2007;71:1311-1315.
[13] M Waner, J Kastenbaum, K Scherer. Hemangiomas of the nose. Arch Facial Plast Surg. 2008;10(5):329-334.
[14] JG McCarthy, LJ Borud, JS Schreiber. Hemangiomas of the nasal tip. Plast Reconstr Surg 2002;109(1):31-40.
[15] SM Warren, MT Longaker, BM Zide. The subunit approach to nasal tip hemangiomas. Plast Reconstr Surg 2002;109(1):25-30.
[16] S Cho, SY Lee, JH Choi, KJ Sung, KC Moon, JK Koh. Treatment of Cyrano angioma with pulsed dye laser. Dermatol Surg 2001;27:670-72.
[17] MJ Denk, N Ajkay, X Yuan, RS Rosenblum, N Freda, WP Magee. Surgical treatment of nasal hemangiomas. Ann Plast Surg 2002;48:489-495.
[18] L Burgos, JC L Gutierrez, AM Andres, JL Encinas, AL Luis, O Suarez, M Dias, Z Ros. Early surgical treatment in nasal tip hemangiomas: 36 cases review. Cir Pediatr 2007;20(2):83-6.
[19] JC van der Meulen, PhM Gilbert, R. Roddi. Early excision of nasal hemangiomas: The L-approach. Plast Reconstr Surg 1993;94(3):465-75.
[20] I Pitanguy, BHB Machado, HR Radwanski, NFG Amorim. Surgical treatment of hemangiomas of the nose. Ann Plast Surg 1996; 36(6):586-92.
[21] K Faguer, A Dompmartin, D Labbe, MT Barrellier, D Leroy, J Theron. Early surgical treatment of Cyrano-nose hemangiomas with Rethi incision. B J Plast Surg. 2002; 55:498-53.

[22] M Hochman, A Mascareno. Management of nasal hemangiomas. Arch. Facial Plast Surg 2005; 7:295-300.

[23] R Simic, A Vlahovic, V Subarevic. Treatment of nasal hemangiomas. Int J Ped Otolar 2009; 73: 1402-1406.

[24] IT Jackson, J Sosa. Excision of nasal tip hemangioma via open rhinoplasty - a skin sparing technique. Eur J Plast Surg 1998;21:265-268.

[25] 25. B Eivazi, HJ Cremer, C Mangold, A Teymoortash, S Wiegand, JAWerner. Hemangiomas of the nasal tip: An approach to a therapeutic challenge. International Journal of Pediatric Otorhinolaryngology 2011; 75: 368–375.

[26] HG Thompson, M Lanigan. The Cyrano nose:a clinical review of hemangioma of the nasal tip. Plast Reconstr Surg 1979;63:155-60.

[27] JS Arneja, H Chim, BA Drolet, AK Gosain. The Cyrano nose:refinements in surgical technique and treatment approach to hemangiomas of the nasal tip. Pl Reconstr Surg 2010;126(4):1291-1299.

[28] C. Leaute-Labreze, E. Dumas de la Roque, T. Hubiche, F. Boralevi. Propranolol for severe hemangiomas of infancy, N. Engl. J. Med 2008; 358: 2649–2651.

[29] AP Zimmermann, S Wiegand, JA Werner, B Eivazi. Propranolol-therapy for infantile haemangiomas: review of literature, Int. J. Pediatr. Otorhinolaryngol. 2010;74: 338–342.

[30] IJ Frieden, AN Haggstrom, Drolet BA et al. Infantile hemangiomas: current knowledge, future directions. Proceedings of a research workshop on infantile hemangiomas. Ped Dermatol 2005;22(5):383-406.

[31] C Hamou, PA Diner, P Dalmonte et al. Nasal tip hemangiomas:guidelines for an early surgical approach. J PL Reconstr Aesth Surg 2010;63:934-939.

[32] EC Siegfried, WJ Keenan, S Al-Jureidini. More on propranolol for hemangiomas of infancy. N Engl J Med. 2008;359(26):2846.

Part 4

Nasal Tip Refinement in Rhinoplasty

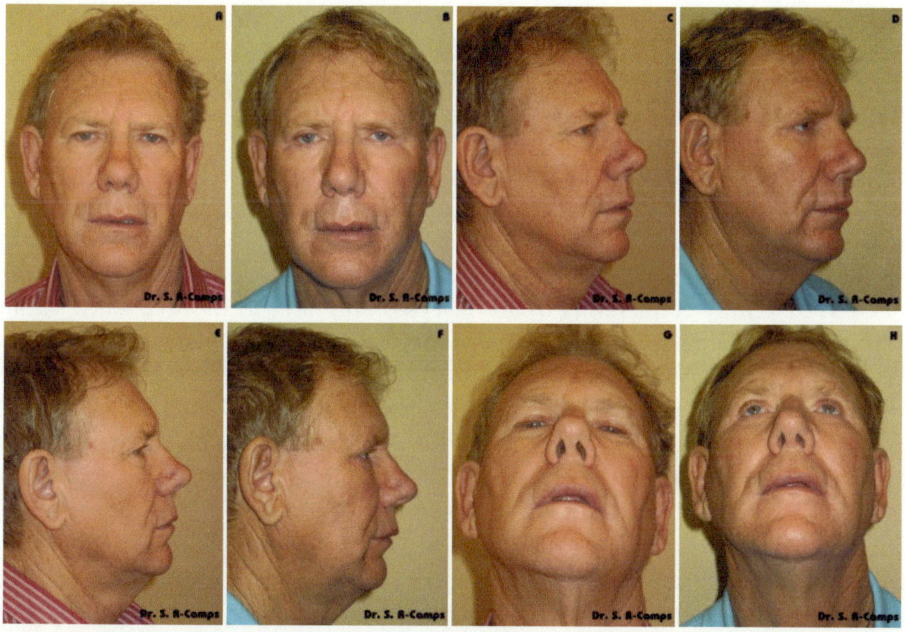

Fig. 7. (A, B, C, D, E, F, G and H) Primary rhinoplasty. Protruding and bulbous tip with very thick skin. Type III resection-reconstruction: Total Resection of the Alar Cartilages, respecting domes. There was no need for temporal fascia given the thickness of the skin. In this particular case, we performed a blepharoplasty simultaneously. Result after 1 year

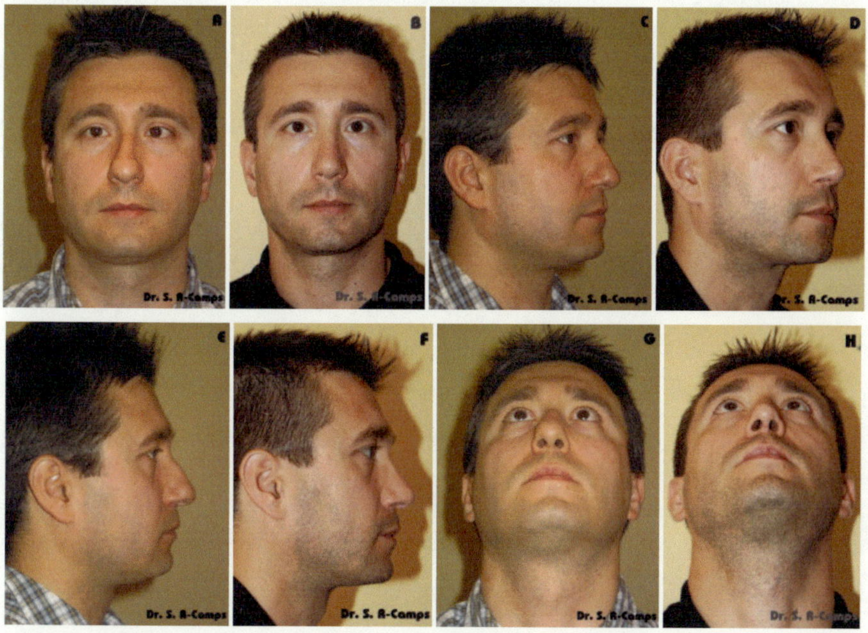

Fig. 8. (A, B, C, D, E, F and H) Primary rhinoplasty. Deviated nose with globulous nasal tip. Type II resection-reconstruction: Total Resection of the Alar Cartilages, including domes. Patch and band of temporal fascia. Killian septoplasty. Result after 1 year

2. Material and methods

"Rhinoplasty is decidedly a very difficult operation although, technically, it seems deceptively easy" (Jack Sheen).

I have operated more than 550 patients with this technique and have over 24 years experience in it (1987–2011) with highly satisfactory results.

In secondary and traumatic Rhinoplasty suits this technique, always Rethi's approach (Open Rhinoplasty), which is especially designed for it. Yet we are increasingly employing it in primary rhinoplasty when the solution for a cartilaginous dome proves difficult with other techniques. We are fully accelerating in this last case and have introduced some variation, as we will go on to explain. Mainly after cancer surgery on the nasal tip, we also have gained experience in nasal reconstruction.

What do I mean when I speak of other nasal tip remodelling techniques? All those known as conventional techniques based on repositioning alar cartilages with grafts removed from ears. Then there are the extreme cases in which the creation of a genuine cartilage scaffolding is easy to detect in many cases when the oedema has disappeared some months later. It is true that these techniques always improve the appearance of the new nasal tip, but it is not hard to detect the presence of peaks and edges corresponding to the grafts taken mainly from the auricular concha. Although I am not in favour of cartilaginous grafts in the nasal tip given the subsequent reabsorption, torsion, asymmetry problems or noted through the skin, I admit I still use some of them to project and define a nasal tip with the shield of Sheen or the champagne glass of Juri, but I no longer use cartilaginous grafts to reconstruct the nasal dome and/or the nasal wings. Other techniques have contributed to the success of the nasal tip treatment, to refine it. Thus, Safian (1930) begins an interesting process which Goldman (1957) would significantly improve, with his vertical dome division (VDD: anterior triangular shape incision of both domes), and Simons and Adamson will popularize it definitively. Lipsett (1959) will modify this technique with multiple parcial thickness incisions in the nasal domes for bending the cartilages.

2.1 The resection

An equilateral and stable nasal base is our main objective. To fulfil this objective, we have classified resections into 5 types (although, in very special cases, it is convenient to make some little combinations between them).

2.1.1 Type I

Complete resection of alar cartilages, including domes and one trunk of the crus medialis.

This is indicated for noses that are long-pointed, have a long columela, and for large and elongated nostrils. Here we introduce some of our technical resources, such as alar wedges, and resecting the crus medialis feet.

2.1.2 Type II

Complete resection of alar cartilages, including domes. This is indicated for noses with a slightly elongated nasal base.

2.1.3 Type III

Total resection of alar cartilages, respecting domes. Applicable to noses whose nasal base is very close to the objective (equilateral nasal base).

2.1.4 Type IV

Total resection of alar cartilages, respecting domes, and leaving two small alar wedges whose latero-caudal length is no longer than 8 mm and is of an arrow-tip shape. Indicated for cases where the nasal base is equilateral.

2.1.5 Type V

Total resection of alar cartilages, respecting domes and approaching the Crus Medialis feet, and suturing domes as high as possible to accomplish projection. Then we remove vestibular wedges, place a Converse stitch, smoothly reduce the soft triangles, release the columela of the base and remove a trunk of the septum depressor muscle. Generally, it is only here where we introduce a septum tutor intercrus to prolong and strengthen the columela projecting the nasal tip. This is indicated for flat and negroid noses with a short columela, separated nasal wings and broad nostrils.

Many times, it is not necessary to use the temporal fascia for covering the crus medialis, because of the thickness of the skin (fig. 7).

(Fig. 9, fig. 10, fig. 11, fig. 12, fig. 13)

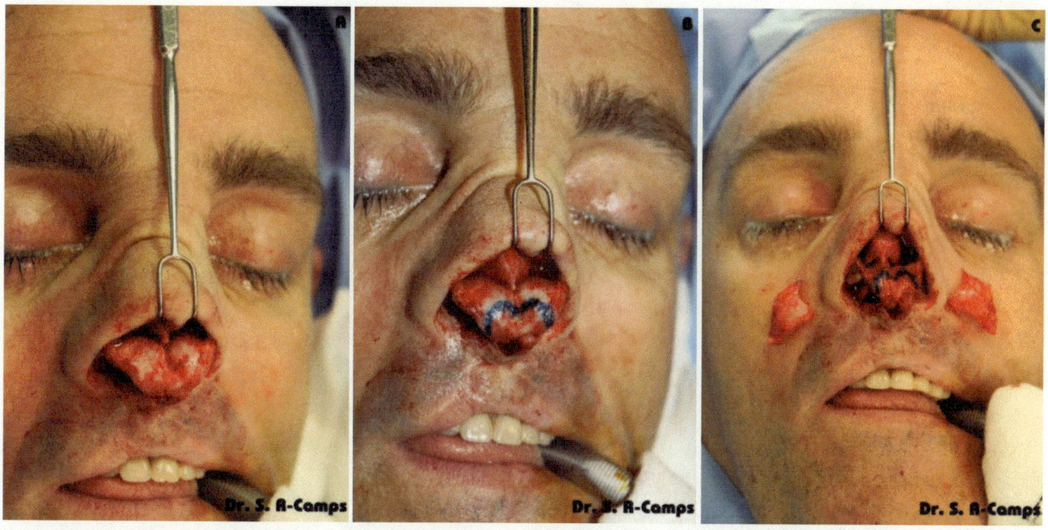

Fig. 9. (A, B and C) Cleft rhinoplasty. Very broad tip with cartilaginous hypertrophy. Type III resection marking: Total Resection of the Alar Cartilages, respecting domes

2.2 The reconstruction

We place two stitches with 5-0 nylon, and conceal the knots, on top of the crus medialis to keep them firmly together. If the approach is complete, sometimes it is not necessary. A patch and/or a band of temporal fascia is placed covering the crus medialis.

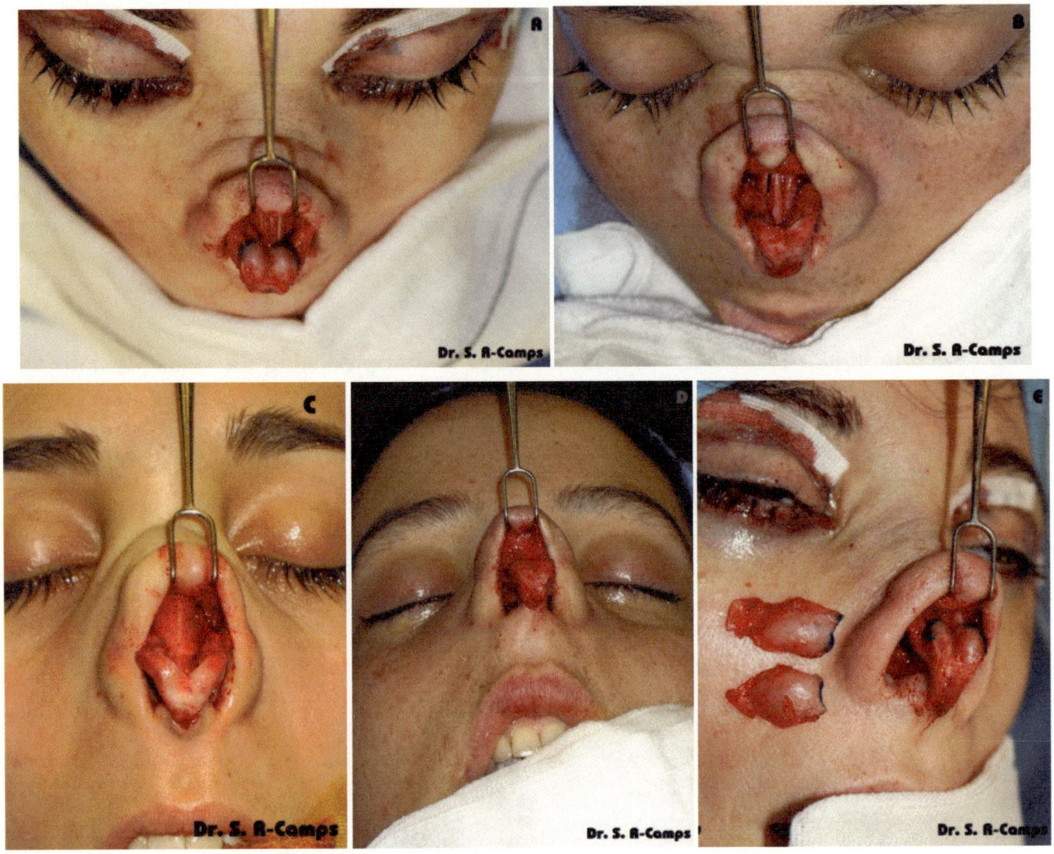

Fig. 10. (A, B, C, D and E) Different resection types

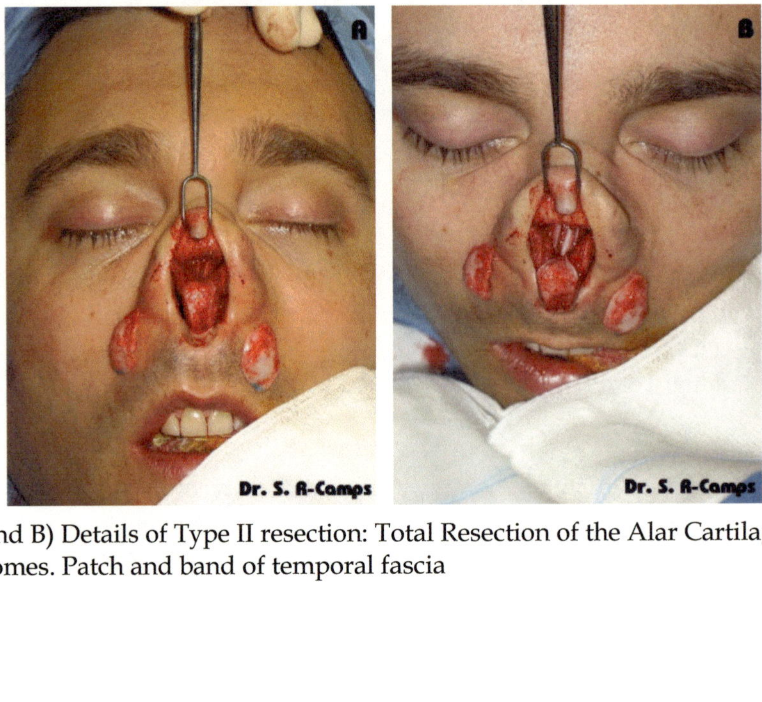

Fig. 11. (A and B) Details of Type II resection: Total Resection of the Alar Cartilages, including domes. Patch and band of temporal fascia

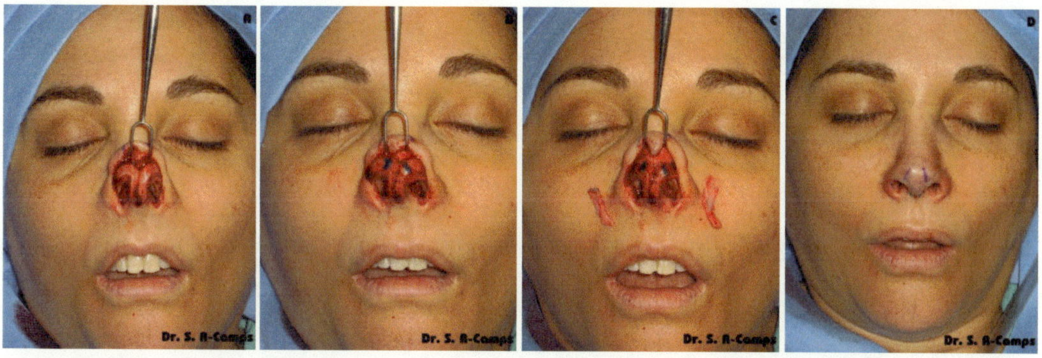

Fig. 12. (A, B, C and D) Secondary rhinoplasty on an extremely broad tip and an inadequate resection. Details of Type II resection and immediate result: Total Resection of the Alar Cartilages, including domes. Patch and band of temporal fascia

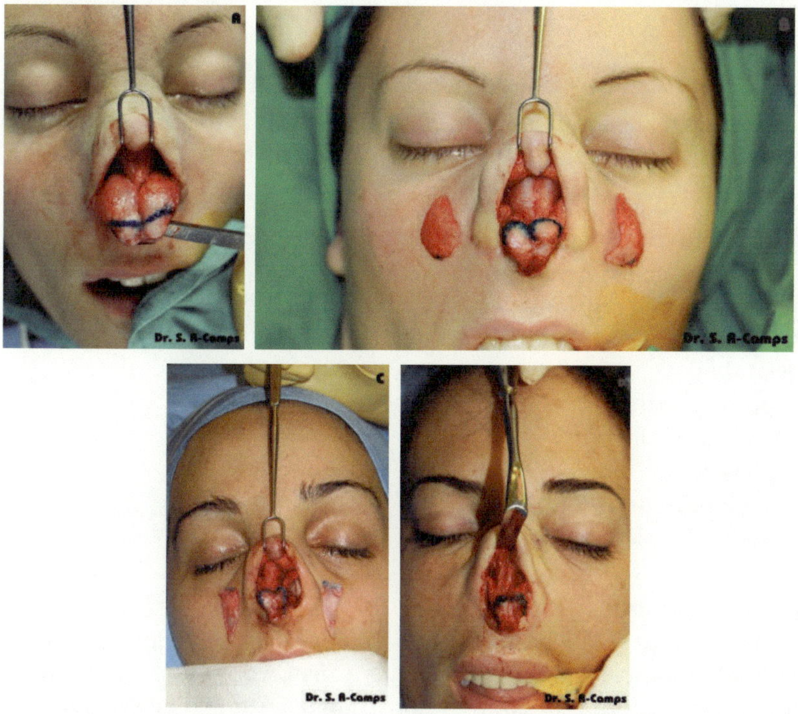

Fig. 13. (A, B, C and D) Different resection types

2.3 The temporal fascia

In 1984, Dr. Guerrerosantos introduced this procedure to increase the dorsal unit of the nose and to fill the naso-frontal angle. We use it for the tip to achieve a firm covering and a beautiful, smooth protection in terms of both sight and touch by joining it as a single plane to the fibroadipose covering to the skin (fig. 14).

We only exclude temporal fascia in those nasal tips with a thick skin, with abundant sebaceous glands and a dense fibroadipose covering.

To avoid a pointed nasal tip, conversely, its placing is essential in Caucasian women and European north-eastern people with delicate and thin skin. There is no problem with a "shrink wrap effect", until nowadays. The technique works very similar in every ethnic group, but we need to use the temporal fascia generally and, however, rarely in black or Asian people because of the thickness of the skin. In every ethnic group we have had no problem with retraction.

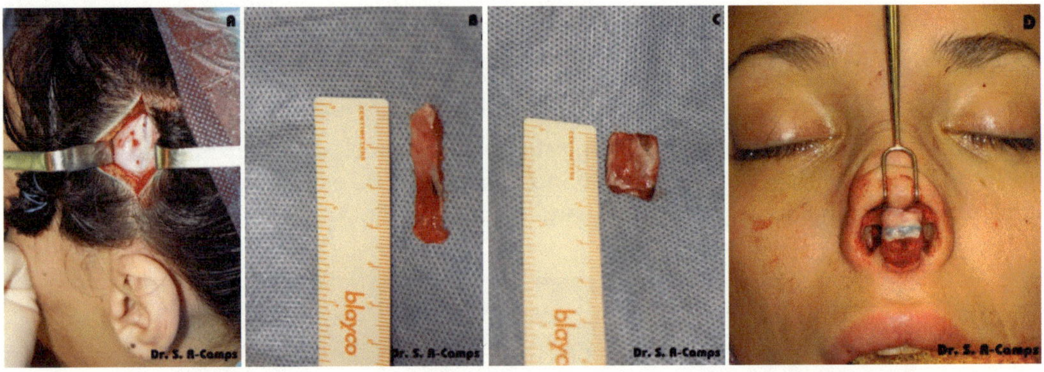

Fig. 14. (A, B, C and D) Details of temporal fascia arranged to be utilized for reconstruction purposes. A fascia seal covering the ends of the crus medialis in a Type II reconstruction

The seal extension will also depend on the thickness of the wings' skin. We place 1 or 2-layered temporal fascia depending on requirements and the resection type, and we sometimes include muscle fibres to provide bulk.

In this way, the anatomy of the new nasal tip and the wings will outwardly to inwardly comprise the following single-body layers:

- Superficial skin
- Fibroadipose covering
- External fibrous lamina
- Temporal fascia
- Internal fibrous lamina
- Internal vestibular skin

2.4 The technical resources

According to the former shape of the nasal base, and to achieve an equilateral nasal base, we use a serie of technical details that enable a firm, consistent base which resists alar collapse during inspiration: reduction of soft triangles (to achieve nostrils with a longer look), resecting a trunk of the septum depressor muscle (to help project the nasal tip and avoid it from moving and lowering when talking and laughing), Converse stitch (to narrow an excessively wide columelar base), releasing the columela (to project the tip, block it and open the naso-labial angle), alar wedges (to bring wings closer together and to reduce the nostrils size), resection or approach of the Crus Medialis Feet (to lower the nasal tip or to project it), tutor intercrus (to strengthen the columela and to project the tip), vestibular wedges (to narrow nostrils), septoplasty (Killian) and/or luxation or cauterisation of the nasal turbinates (to ensure the respiratory tract function and to be able to perform the technique without the possibility of collapse), and filling the nasolabial angle with resected remains (fig. 15) (to obtain beauty between the lip and the nasal base).

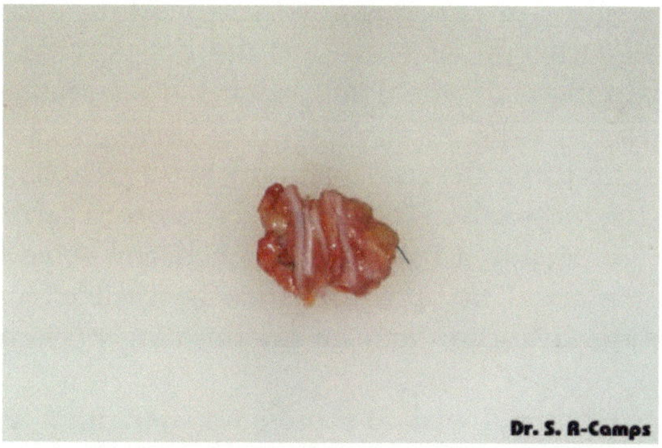

Fig. 15. Details of removed and sutured alar cartilages prepared to be introduced into the naso-labial angle for the purpose of opening it

As regards the septum and nasal turbinates being responsible for a correct respiratory tract, we have highlighted that many of the bulges in the cartilaginous dome of the tip are due to natural compensation caused by a deviation of the septum and/or to a hypertrophy of the turbinates. If we perform the total resection of alar cartilages technique with their domes without having previously treated any pathology in the septum and turbinates, then we will cause nasal respiratory insufficiency with spontaneous collapse and/or during inhalation. If, on the other hand, the septum and turbinates are normal, we should not come across complications of any kind of either a functional or an aesthetic type when undertaking a total resection of the cartilaginous dome of the nasal tip.

2.5 The postoperative period

The postoperative period does not differ much with our technique from that of other techniques (if anything, recuperation is shorter). However, we have to maintain the vestibular cotton pads pushing the domes for 4-5 days (fig. 16). A plaster splint remains in place for 7 days, and a double layer of Steri-Strip^R is used for 7 additional days.

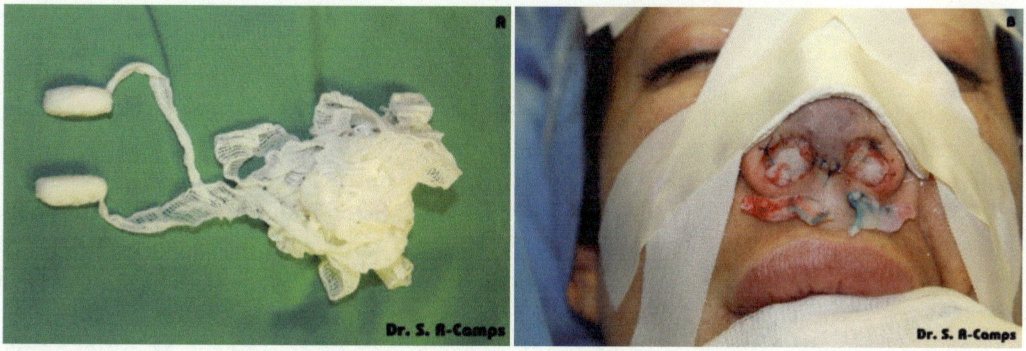

Fig. 16. (A and B) Details of prepared cotton pads of sufficient length to be positioned to push the vestibular skin from the dome and to ensure a compact union with the fascia and tip skin

3. Results

Judging from our patients' degree of satisfaction, the results obtained since 1987 to date in 2011, range from very good to excellent. Other nasal tip reconstruction techniques performed with complex cartilaginous structures did not provide us with the best results because a "surgical tip" emerged when the oedema disappeared, with traces of barely admissible tips and edges.
We reconstruct the nasal tip using the cartilages we have available, and if they do not serve this purpose, we resect them directly. We very rarely resort to cartilaginous grafts since we adopted our technique. Personally, I reached the conclusion some time ago of NOT using cartilaginous grafts in the nasal tip, provided this is feasible, for ultimate problems of displacement, reabsorption, distortion and an unappealing presentation in terms of sight and touch.
Despite what I have stated herein, I wish to express my maximum respect and admiration to all the Rhinoplasty Masters from whom I have learnt.
We have had no problems with the ever-feared alar collapse, which is most certainly due to other factors such as an excessive resection of the triangular cartilages, a vestibular valve lesion without correcting a significant deviation of the septum during surgery, or hypertrophic turbinates which could contribute to or even cause nasal respiratory failure with a uni or a bilateral collapse. Regarding complications, there is nothing particular to highlight in either aesthetic or functional terms.

4. Discussion

I realised that this technique was controversial, from the beginning, and that our Rhinoplasty Masters did no advice an excessive resection of alar cartilages, but preferred to maintain a cartilage band of a width of no less than 3-5 mm in the latero-caudal sense to avoid alar collapse. However, by following the steps of our technique and by maintaining its main objective (an equilateral, solid nasal base with a firm, yet soft nasal tip in terms of sight and touch, with no cartilaginous remains in view) I have verified and demonstrated that this may be avoided.
Nonetheless, all this involves experience in rhinoplasty and a totally accurate technique. It proves a most useful technique, but to be used only in extremely difficult nasal tip cases.

5. Conclusion

My new technique has posed no problems when well indicated, diagnosed and performed, and has matured sufficiently over time in casuistry.
Finally, the nasal tip becomes as firm and consistent, or more, than prior to surgery. Its five anatomical layers retract in a uniform fashion without distortions. To the touch, it is solid yet smooth and, aesthetically, it offers a beautiful result. Only a biopsy would enable us to verify the state of the stratification, but it is complicated proposing this to a patient who is satisfied with his or her nose, and we are all aware of the possible negative consequences of extracting a cylinder of tissue with the more than likely alteration to the vectorial system and to shape. It would be rather like requesting a "structural sampling" in a cathedral vault to learn the characteristics or state of its materials. Thus, our colleagues should trust in the technique thanks to its results.

The most difficult plastic surgery operation is undoubtedly rhinoplasty and, within it, nasal tip cases are extremely difficult. Nonetheless, the operation is the most appealing and fascinating of our speciality, but great care must be taken while performing it.
I literally cite: ... *"The author must be congratulated for his work, and be honoured and highly commended for the results obtained. This study is unique and it offers excellent results"... "Indeed, these results will convince many of us in practicing these aggressive resections"...*
"The complete and permanent removal of what Mother Nature has designed requires the broadest experience, competence and an aesthetic feel by a Master Craftsman in a procedure that permits a minor error, or absolutely none. I therefore completely agree with the author that this procedure cannot be generally applied to all nasal tip operations, and that it is not suitable for enthusiastic beginners in surgery who lack both experience and aesthetic criteria"... "It is likely that the author has found temporal fascia an ideal substitute after totally resecting alar cartilages. (Dr. Neeta Patel, in her commentary on this technique in the Aesthetic Plastic Surgery Journal. January 2009).
Furthermore: *"Dr. Rodríguez-Camps' contribution makes this nasal tip technique most interesting for difficult cases"...*
"We are well aware that the nasal tip is one of the most difficult parts of Rhinoplasty, and that all of us have the technique that provides the best results available; but we also know that some rhinoplasty cases are very difficult to solve. Dr. Rodríguez-Camps' technique of totally removing alar cartilages and then introducing temporal fascia is novel and interesting"... "Needless to say, the results obtained by Dr. Rodríguez-Camps are excellent and we are enthusiastic about using this nasal aesthetic technique" (Dr. Guerrerosantos in his commentary on the technique in Cirugía Plástica Iberolatinoamericana. Jan.-Feb.-March 2010).
We conclude that when it seemed that everything had been described, and that the results depended only on our hands, something new and fresh appears: "The Total Resection of the Alar Cartilages and Temporal Fascia Technique".

6. References

Burget G, M.D. & Menick F, M.D.: Aesthetic Reconstruction of the Nose. First Edition. Mosby. 1994.

Converse J, M.D.: Reconstructive Plastic Surgery. Second Edition. W. B. Saunders Company. Philadelphia, London, Toronto. Vol. 2 Chapter 29, 1040-1281. 1977.

Ezquerra Carrera F., Sainz-Arregui J. & Berrazueta Fernández M. J.: La Rinoplastia No Basica Primaria. Cir. Plast. Iberlatinamer. Vol. 27 – N0. 1. January-February-March 2001. Pages 45-54.

Goldman IB.: Eye Ear Nose Throat Mon, 1957 Dec; 36 (12):742-3.

Guerrerosantos, J.: Temporoparietal Free Fascia Grafts in Rhinoplasty. Plastic and Reconstructive Surgery. Vol. 74. Issue 4. pag. 465-474. October 1984.

Jack P. Gunter, M.D., Rod J. Rohrich, M.D. & William P. Adams, Jr. M.D.: Dallas Rhinoplasty. Nasal Surgery by the Masters. Second Edition. Quality Medical Publishing, Inc. St. Louis, Missouri. Vol. I, 303-590. 2007.

Juri J, M.D., Juri C, M.D., Grilli D, M.D., Zeaiter MC, M.D. & Belmont J, M.D.: Correction of the Secondary Nasal Tip. Annals of Plastic Surgery. Vol. 16. N0. 4. 322-332. April 1986.

Lipsett EM.: A new approach surgery of the lower cartilaginous vault. AMA Arch Otolaryngol, 1959 Jul; 70(1): 42-7.

Meyer R.: Secondary and Functional Rhinoplasty. The Difficult Nose. First Edition. Grune & Stratton, Inc. Orlando, Florida. 1988.

Peck G, M.D. Techniques in Aesthetic Rhinoplasty. First Edition. Gower Medical Publishing Ltd. New York, NY, U.S.A. 1984.

Rodriguez-Camps S: Secondary Rhinoplasty in Cleft Nose. Rethi Technique. XX Spanish National Plastic, Reconstructive and Aesthetic Surgery Society (SECPRE) Meeting. Video Presentation. León, Spain. October, 1989.

Rodriguez-Camps S: Nasal Reconstruction after Mohs Micrographic Surgery. Poster. Spanish National Reconstructive, Aesthetic and Plastic Surgery Society (SECPRE) Congress. Valladolid, Spain. June, 1994.

Rodriguez-Camps S: Reconstrucción Nasal tras Cirugía Micrográfica de Mohs. Cir Plast Iberolatinoamer. Vol. XXI, no.3, 215-223, 1995.

Rodriguez-Camps S: Total Reconstructive Rhinoplasty with the medial forehead flap. VIII Spanish National Reconstructive, Aesthetic and Plastic Surgery Society (SECPRE) Congress. Video Presentation. Santiago de Compostela, Spain. June, 1995.

Rodriguez-Camps S: Nose Reconstruction with medial forehead flap after Mohs Surgery. International Video-Journal of Plastic and Aesthetic Surgery. Vol. 2, nº 3, December 1995.

Rodriguez-Camps S: Aesthetic Rhinoplasty under local anaesthesia without sedation. XXXI Spanish National Reconstructive, Aesthetic and Plastic Surgery Society (SECPRE) Congress. Video Presentation. Madrid, Spain. September, 1996.

Rodriguez-Camps S: Augmentative Rhinoplasty with auricular cartilage. Spanish National Reconstructive, Aesthetic and Plastic Surgery Society (SECPRE) Congress. Barcelona, Spain. April, 1997.

Rodriguez-Camps S: Relapsing Basal Cell Ephithelioma of the nasal tip. Resection. Two-stage reconstruction with a frontal flap. Nasal Plastic surgery Symposium, tribute to Dr. Vilar-Sancho. The Ramón y Cajal Hospital, Madrid, Spain. February, 1998.

Rodriguez-Camps S: Augmentative Rhinoplasty with an Auricular Gibbus. Aesth Plast Surg. Vol.22. nº. 3.196-205, 1998.

Rodriguez-Camps S: Miscellaneous Rhinoplasty: Primary and Secondary. XXXIV Spanish National Reconstructive, Aesthetic and Plastic Surgery Society (SECPRE) Congress. Marbella, Spain. April, 1999.

Rodriguez-Camps S: Rhinoplasty: Primary, Secondary and Reconstructive. II Plastic, Reconstructive and Aesthetic Surgery Society Meeting of the Valencian Community (SCPRECV). Alicante, Spain. February, 2000.

Rodriguez-Camps S: Nasal Reconstruction After Epithelioma. Aesth Plastic Surg. Vol. 25. No. 4:273-277. July-August 2001.

Rodriguez-Camps S: Aesthetic Nasal Reconstruction from the Oficial Book of the XXXVII Spanish National Reconstructive, Aesthetic and Plastic Surgery Society (SECPRE) Congress. Rhinoplasty, Chapter 11. Oviedo, Spain. June, 2002.

Rodriguez-Camps S: Rhinoplasty. The Aesthetic Tip-Columela-Lip Unit. XV Latin American Federation of Plastic Surgery Congress (FILACP) and XXXIX Spanish National Reconstructive, Aesthetic and Plastic Surgery Society (SECPRE) Congress. Seville, Spain. May, 2004.

Rodriguez-Camps S: Rhinoplasty: Nasal Base. V Plastic, Reconstructive and Aesthetic Surgery Society Meeting of the Valencian Community (SCPRECV). General University Hospital, Alicante, Spain. November, 2004.

Rodriguez-Camps S: Nasal Reconstruction. VI National Reconstructive, Aesthetic and Plastic Surgery Society Meeting of the Valencian Community (SCPRECV). Valencia, Spain. October, 2005.

Rodriguez-Camps S: Closed Rhinoplasty. Teaching Course on National Reconstructive, Aesthetic and Plastic Surgery. School of Medicine. University of Barcelona, Spain. November, 2005.

Rodriguez-Camps S: Secondary Rhinoplasty: Our procedure. Total Resection of the Alar Cartilages and Domes with a Temporal Fascia Stamp on the Tip. XLI Spanish National Reconstructive, Aesthetic and Plastic Surgery Society (SECPRE) Congress. Paper. Pamplona, Spain. May, 2006.

Rodriguez-Camps S: Nasal Reconstruction. VII Reconstructive, Aesthetic and Plastic Society Meeting of the Valencian Community (SCPRECV) Meeting. Alzira, Valencia, Spain. October, 2006.

Rodriguez-Camps S: Reconstructive Rhinoplasty. Teaching Course on Reconstructive, Aesthetic and Plastic Surgery. School of Medicine. University of Barcelona, Spain. November, 2006.

Rodriguez-Camps S: Rhinoplasty. The Difficult Nasal Tip: Total Resection of the Alar Cartilages. XIX Congress of the International Society of Aesthetic Plastic Surgery, (ISAPS). Panelist. Melbourne, Australia. February, 2008.

Rodriguez-Camps S: Rhinoplasty. The Difficult Nasal Tip: Total Resection of the Alar Cartilages. Aesth. Plast. Surg. Vol. 33. No. 1. 72-83. January 2009.

Rodriguez-Camps S: Una nueva técnica para el tratamiento de la punta nasal difícil. Experiencia personal de 22 años (1987-2009). Cirugía Plástica Ibero-latinoamericana Journal. Cir. Plast. Iberolatinoam. Vol. 36. No. 1. Pages 3-12. January-February-March 2010.

Rodriguez-Camps S: New technique to treat a very difficult nasal tip. Total resection of the Alar Cartliages and Temporal Fascia Covering XLV Spanish National Reconstructive, Aesthetic and Plastic Surgery Society (SECPRE) Congress. Gerona, Spain. May, 2010.

Rodriguez-Camps S: Demostrating the Total Resection of the Alar Cartilages and Temporal Fascia Technique on a corpse as part of the VI Theoretical-Practical Course on Anatomical Disection organized by the Spanish Association of Aesthetic Plastic Surgery (AECEP). I Course on Rhinoplasty and Facial Implants. Department of Human Anatomy and Embryology II, School of Medicine at the Complutense University of Madrid. Madrid, Spain. July 2010.

Rodriguez-Camps S: Un paso adelante en Rinoplastia: Técnica de Resección Total de los Cartílagos Alares y Fascia Temporal. Spanish Association of Aesthetic Plastic Surgery Journal (AECEP). N°. 12. Pages 13-24. July-December 2010.

Sheen J.: Aesthetic Rhinoplasty. Second Edition. The C.V. Mosby Company. Saint Louis 1978.

Soria, J.H., Pintos, J.C., Conde, C.G. & Losardo, R.J.: Sobrepunta Nasal como Expresión de una Comunicación Septal. Cir.Plast. Iberolatinoam. Vol.35 n°. 4. October–

November–December 2009. Pages 243-248. Commentary on the work: Dr. Rodríguez-Camps, S.

Tardy M. E. Jr., M.D.: Surgical Anatomy of the Nose. First Edition. Raven Press, Ltd. New York, USA. 1990.

Wolfgang Gubisch, M.D.: Overresection of the Lower Lateral Cartilages: A Common Conceptual Mistake with Functional and Aesthetic Consequences. Aesth. Plast. Surg. 33:6-13 (2009).

Part 5

Minimally Invasive Techniques

9

Minimally Invasive Approach for Rhinoplasty

S. Cohen
Plastic and Aesthetic Surgery, Private Clinic, Ramat Gan
Israel

1. Introduction

The nose, the most prominent aesthetic feature in the facial profile, is a three-dimensional, intricate trapezoid solid, encompassing the external bony and cartilaginous vault with an overlying skin cover and internal cavities. Through their intricate structural interdependency, these topographic features contribute both to form and function. Given its central location in the midface, the nose interrelates with the adjacent structures through juxtaposition, ultimately giving rise to the overall size, shape, and aesthetics of the nose.

Ideal facial and nasal forms have been depicted from ancient Egyptian hieroglyphics to the Renaissance era. These cannons dictated what is most desirable and possibly achievable. Correction of aesthetic nasal deformities date back to India in 600 BC by Sushruta Samhita. Since then, there has been a long evolution of techniques. Different surgical approaches have been advocated, each with its inherent advantages and liabilities. Optimal rhinosculpturing outcomes are not achieved merely as a consequence of the access route but rather rely on a precise execution of a technique that addresses the deformity.

Science and art are inseparable in rhinoplasty. Gratifying results performed by surgical intervention or minimally invasive procedures require systematic analysis of the anatomic variables, adherence to structured strategy, artistic perception, and precise manipulation. It is a well known tenet to all surgical endeavors that a sound knowledge of anatomy is requisite and the reader is advised to refer to a comprehensive review of *Surgical anatomy of the nose*, by O'Neal, et al. 1996 (1).

2. Nasal aesthetics

Balance, harmony and symmetry are essential elements of beauty; thus, a thorough nasal and facial analysis in frontal, lateral, and basal views is of paramount importance in achieving state-of-the-art results in rhinoplasty.

Although a complete description of nasal analysis is beyond the scope of this article, certain fundamental considerations merit discussion.

In the frontal view, assessment of balance is achieved by dividing the face into horizontal thirds (trichion to glabella, glabella to subnasale, and subnasale to menton), and vertical fifths. The nose should represent one-third of the length of the face and one-fifth, the width (Figure 1). The ideal shape of the nose is outlined by two slightly curved divergent lines extending from the medial brows to the tip-defining points. The width of the alar base is equal to the intercanthal distance (Figure 1). The width of the nasal base comprises approximately 70% to 80% of the alar base.

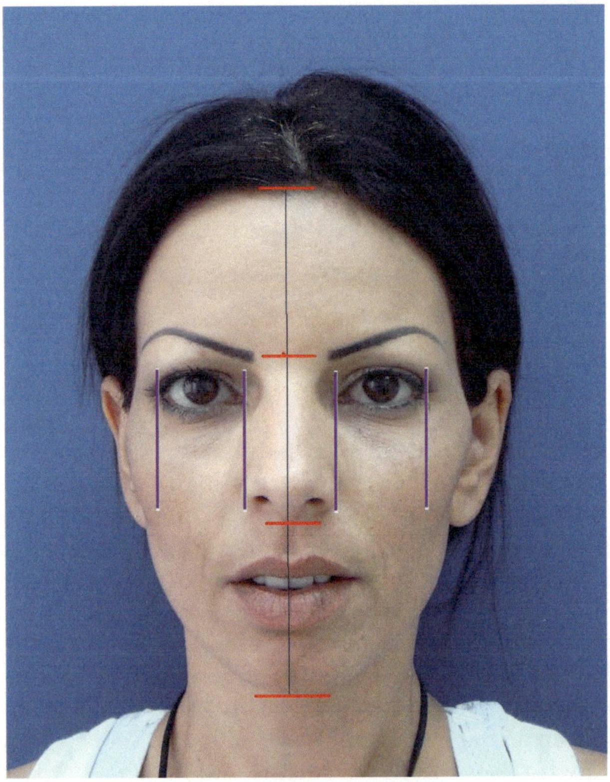

Fig. 1. The face is divided into thirds by horizontal lines drawn from the hair line, glabella, subnasale and menton. The nose should represent one-third of the length of the face and one-fifth of its width. Alar base is equal to the intercanthal distance

In the lateral view, important parameters include nasal length, tip rotation, tip projection and dorsal contour. Nasal length (or dorsal length) is determined by the vertical distance from the nasion (root of the nose overlying the nasofrontal suture) to the tip-defining point. Tip rotation is equivalent to the nasolabial angle, which measures the rotation of the nasal base from the upper lip. In women, it is 95^0 to 105^0. In men, it is 90^0 to 95^0 (Figure 2). Nasal tip projection is commonly assessed by Goode's method (2). Goode defines ideal nasal projection (measured from the alar crease to the tip-defining point) as 0.55 to 0.60 in relation to the dorsal length. Assessment of the dorsal contour should identify any concavity, convexity or irregularity. In women, the aesthetic nasal dorsum lies approximately 2 mm behind and parallel to a line from the nasofrontal angle to the tip, with a slight supratip break offsetting the nasal tip from the dorsum. In men, the dorsum should be slightly higher and a subtle convexity is typical.

The relationship of the ala and columella is likewise assessed on profile. Acceptable columellar show is between 2 mm to 4 mm.

On profile view, one should be acquainted with the Powell and Humphrey's aesthetic angles applied in facial analysis (2). Of these, nasofrontal and nasofacial angles should be carefully assessed. As an angle interrelates two juxtaposed lines, changing the inclination of one line will consequently alter the perceived overall proportions, and in particular, the apparent nasal length.

The nasofrontal angle (the angle formed between the forehead inclination and the nasal dorsum) is 130±7 degrees in men and 134±7 degrees in women (Figure 3). A deep nasofrontal angle contributes to the illusion of a short nose (and apparent overprojection), and a shallow nasofrontal angle adds apparent length to the nose. The nasofacial angle refers to the inclination between the nasal dorsum and the frontal plane (defined as a line from the nasion to the pogonion, the most prominent anterior projection of the chin). It is 36^0 in men and 34^0 in women.

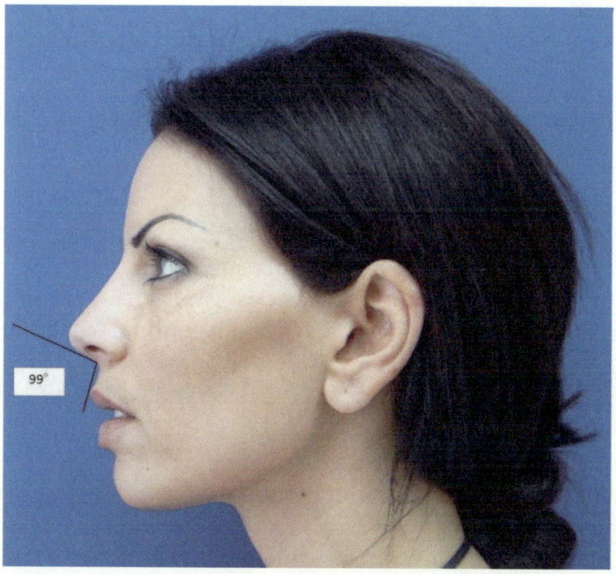

Fig. 2. Tip rotation is determined by the nasolabial angle. In women, it is 95-105^0; in men, it is 90-95^0

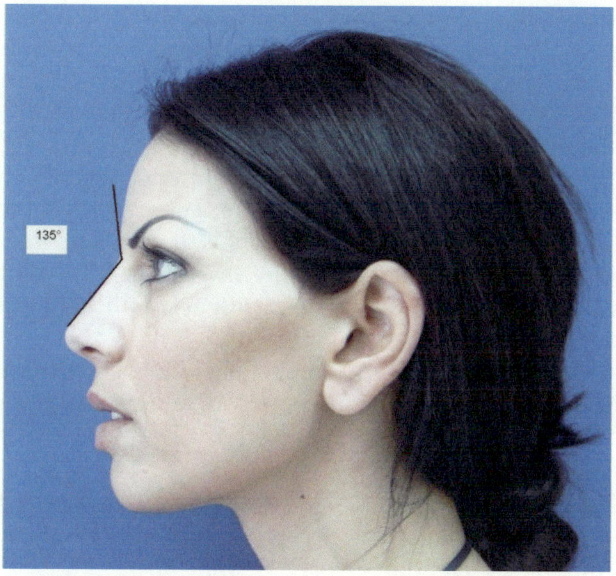

Fig. 3. Nasofrontal angle in women is 134±7^0; in men, it is 130±7^0

On base view, attention should be paid to symmetry, triangularity, columella-to-labial ratio, and width of the alar base. The nasal base should appear as an isosceles triangle with the upper third representing the tip lobule and the lower two-thirds corresponding to the columella.

As facial structures interrelate through juxtaposition, ultimately altered proportions of one part affect the perceived aesthetic appearance of adjacent parts. Nasal aesthetic appearance is likewise influenced by interrelated structures of the chin, forehead and premaxilla, and these should be individually analyzed.

Chin projection is assessed by a perpendicular line drawn between the Frankfurt horizontal line (FHL, a line connecting the superior aspect of the tragus to the infraorbital rim) and nasion. This perpendicular line should intersect the pogonion at 0±2 mm. Alternatively, a perpendicular line from FHL through subnasale should intersect the pogonion 3±3 mm posterior to the line. An underprojected chin may lead to the perception of an overprojected nose and *vice versa*. A flat forehead gives the illusion of increased nose length (3).

As the premaxilla and the pyriform aperture serve as scaffolding for the nasal pyramid, anterior or posterior displacement of these anatomic landmarks may give the illusion of overprojection or retruded nasal profile, respectively. Deficiency of the premaxilla may present as a congenital deformity. Maxilla alveolar hypoplasia along with midfacial retrusion may be congenital or arise as part of the normal aging process (4). Loss of the underlying nasal support imparts an impression of a relative lengthening and retrusion to the aging nose (4)

Different aesthetic facial proportions exist among different faces and ethnicities. Nevertheless, similar concepts of beauty exist among people of various cultural backgrounds in cross-cultural studies (5). Accepted cultural standards and essential elements of beauty are the ultimate goals regardless of the patient's ethnic descent or race.

3. Minimally invasive techniques in rhinoplasty

During the last two decades, minimally invasive facial aesthetic procedures have gained widespread popularity. According to the American Society for Aesthetic Plastic Surgery (ASAPS), the annual number of nonsurgical cosmetic procedures increased by 228% from 1997 to 2010, and in 2010, nonsurgical procedures accounted for 83% of the aesthetic procedures performed overall (6).

While botulinum toxin injection tops the ASAPS's annual list as the most commonly performed cosmetic procedure since 2000, soft tissue augmentation procedures accounted for more than 15% of the procedures performed in 2010. Breakdown by filler type of soft tissue augmentation procedures reported by the ASAPS in 2010 indicated that calcium hydroxylapatite (CaHA) is the second most frequently used filler following hyaluronic acid (HA) filler derivatives.

Purported advantages over traditional surgeries include lack of scars, minimal down-time, less pain, and lower cost. The nose is amenable to a variety of minimally invasive techniques.

3.1 Indications

Minimally invasive nonsurgical techniques in rhinoplasty allow for gratifying results in a variety of indications, including augmentation type primary rhinoplasty(rhinosculpturing), correction of post-rhinoplasty contour defects, treating the aging nose, dealing with the ethnic nose and ameliorating/ reversing selected functional nasal impairments.

4. Augmentation type rhinosculpture

Augmentation type, minimally invasive techniques might be utilized to correct both aesthetic and functional nasal deformities (i.e., internal valve collapse). Architectural deficiencies or imperfections necessitating augmentation type procedures can be systematically categorized by dividing the nose and nasal skeleton into thirds:

1. Upper-third - low radix (root of the nose), widened bony pyramid, bony contour irregularities.
2. Middle-third - low dorsum, dorsal contour irregularities, saddle nose deformity.
3. Lower-third - inadequate tip projection, underrotated tip, retracted columella.

1. Upper-third

Low radix. The radix corresponds to the nasofrontal groove at a level approximately between the supratarsal fold and the upper lash margin on straight gaze, and approximately 9-14 mm anterior to the corneal projection. When the radix begins lower than the upper lash margin, nasal length is shorter and the nasal base size appears to be larger. By augmenting a low radix, the nasofrontal angle is displaced cephalically, increasing the distance from nasion to the tip-defining point. This creates the perception of a larger appearing nose, improves the apparent overprojected tip, and gives rise to a more balanced and proportional aesthetic appearance.

Widened bony pyramid. The width of the bony vault should be analyzed both at the bony base and at the dorsal ridge. Ideal width varies from individual to individual and is influenced by the overall facial width, nasal length and projection, and by skin thickness. Apparent widening of the bony pyramid might be secondary to loss of height and light reflex from the nasal dorsum. In the case of a widened bony pyramid, augmentation of the central bony pyramid may effectively narrow the perceived width.

Bony contour irregularities. These irregularities can be de-emphasized and unsightly depressions can be eliminated or reduced.

2. Middle-third

Low dorsum. Dorsal height is assessed on profile view. Low dorsum refers to a dorsum that lies more than 2 mm behind and parallel to a line from the nasofrontal angle to the tip-defining point, and presents primarily as a congenital deformity, a consequence of previous trauma or as a common characteristic of the ethnic nose, such as the platyrrhine and the African American nose. Augmentation of a low dorsum is performed by using a dorsal graft or via a minimally invasive technique.

Saddle nose deformity. This deformity refers to an abnormally concave nasal dorsum in profile. Predisposing factors include previous trauma, rhinoplastic surgery (overresection of the septum, excessive dorsal hump resection), infectious disease (i.e., syphilis, leprosy), inflammatory disease (i.e., Wegener granulomatosis), neoplastic causes and platyrrhine nasal structure. Associated nasal defects commonly seen include cephalic tip rotation, middle vault collapse, and loss of tip support. In appropriately selected cases, correction for saddle deformity can be achieved by nasal dorsum augmentation alone, whereas more severe deformities mandate structural realignment with conventional approaches.

3. Lower-third

Inadequate tip projection. Tip projection is conventionally assessed by measuring the distance of the tip-defining point from a facial parameter (i.e., nasion, alar crease) (7,8).

However, in some cases, the nasal bases are large, yet the tip cartilages have poor projection. An alternative functional definition is proposed by Constantian (9). A tip with inadequate projection is defined as any tip that does not project to the level of the septal angle (identified in the supratip as the edge of the dorsal septal angle). An underprojected tip generates the illusion of a dorsal pseudo-hump in the supratip region, secondary to lack of support and discontinuity in the supratip-lobule region. Augmentation of the nasal tip and supratip lobule region can affectively support and project the tip and disguise discontinuity in the caudal dorsum.

Underrotated tip. As alluded to previously, the perceived degree of tip rotation is defined by the nasolabial angle. Desired tip rotation is influenced by gender and by the patient's height (inversely proportional). In women, it is 95 to 105 degrees, whereas a more acute angle of approximately 90 degrees is considered aesthetic in men. Cephalic or caudal positioning of the tip leads to corresponding change in the nasal length, tip rotation and columellar inclination. An overly obtuse nasolabial angle makes the nose appear short, whereas the converse adds apparent length. By augmenting a ptotic tip, the tip-defining point is displaced cephalically so the distance between nasion to the tip-defining point is reduced, thus making the nose appear shorter and aesthetically projected. Augmentation of the anterior nasal spine of the maxillary bone located at the central part of the nasal base opens the nasolabial angle and rotates the tip cephalically.

5. Post-rhinoplasty deformities

Postoperative rhinoplasty complications range from 8% to 15% (10) and result primarily from failure to maintain adequate cartilaginous and bony structural support. Aesthetic deformities often have functional implications and reflect the interdependency of form and function.

Detailed systematic analysis of each of the structural and functional anatomic variables is of utmost importance to determine the correct diagnosis and to properly select a treatment plan. Postoperative complications that result from overresection/overcorrection following overzealous surgery are often amenable to augmentation techniques and will be presented in accordance to the nasal thirds:

1. Upper-third (nasion to rhinion) - low radix, low dorsum, dorsal irregularities, skeletal deformities.
2. Middle-third – inverted V deformity, supratip deformity, saddle nose deformity.
3. Lower-third – external valve incompetence, loss of tip support.

1. Upper-third

Dorsal irregularities result from unsmoothed residual bony or cartilaginous ("mid-dorsal notch") fragments following hump removal. Poorly performed osteotomies result in palpable **skeletal deformities**. These include "open roof" deformity, "step off´ deformities and Rocker deformity. Rocker deformity occurs when medial osteotomy is taken too high into the thick frontal bone. Consequently, the superior aspect of the osteotomized nasal bone projects or "rocks" laterally. By augmentation of these untoward postrhinoplasty sequelae, these deformities are de-emphasized or even eliminated. Likewise, an overresected dorsum or low radix, otherwise necessitating dorsal or radix grafts, can be successfully augmented using minimally invasive procedures.

2. Middle-third

Inverted V deformity refers to inferomedial collapse of the upper lateral cartilage (ULC) consequent to inadequate support of the ULC following overresection of the cartilaginous roof during hump removal. At its caudal end, the ULC ideally forms an angle of 10 to 15 degrees with the septum near the anterior-septal angle. This region is defined as the internal nasal valve and requires patency for normal airway.
When the middle vault collapses towards the anterior septal edge, internal nasal valve collapse ensues, resulting in nasal airway obstruction and inverted V deformity.
Alignment of the internal valve area can improve the nasal airway and disguise the accompanying aesthetic deformity, thus targeting both form and function. Traditionally, correction of internal valve incompetence is accomplished by placing spreader grafts, either unilaterally or bilaterally, that serve as spacer grafts between the dorsal septum and upper lateral cartilage during rhinoplasty.
Supratip deformity (Polly beak) refers to postoperative fullness of the supratip and a blunt tip lobular poorly differentiated from the dorsum. Inadequate tip support and over-resection of the bony hump or cartilage [e.g., dorsal septum, dome or lower lateral cartilage (LLC)] are etiologies that are amenable to augmentation by minimally invasive techniques, with injection to appropriate areas simulating the effect of a columellar strut and dorsal grafts.

3. Lower-third

External valve incompetence. The external nasal valve refers to the area delineated by the cutaneous and skeletal support of the mobile alar wall. Overresection of the lateral crus can lead to collapse of the external valve with negative pressure of respiration, and consequent nasal airway obstruction. Alar retraction, pinching, bossae and tip asymmetry are accompanying changes. Augmentations of the inadequate skeletal support can stabilize the external valve and ameliorate nasal obstruction. Traditionally, it is accomplished by alar batten grafts. The size and precise placement of this augmentation are dependent upon the corrections needed to be performed.
Loss of tip support. One of the most common iatrogenic complications of rhinoplasty is loss of tip support secondary to interrupted major or minor tip support mechanisms. Major support mechanisms include the interlocking attachment of ULC and LLC, LLC size, shape and length, and the medial crural foot plate attachments to caudal septum. Minor support mechanisms are the cartilaginous and membranous septum, the interdomal ligament (fibrous connective tissue attachment between the medial and middle crura) and LLC attachment to the skin.
Recognition of the effects of incisions and resections during rhinoplasty that violate these support mechanisms should be thoroughly appreciated. The exact causes of loss of support should be identified and countered. Commonly, cartilage grafts are used for augmentation to establish acceptable contours: alar batten grafts are used to support the alar rims, strut grafts stabilize the medial crura, and tip grafts support and contour the tip. Once identified, loss of tip support can be overcome via invasive or minimally invasive augmentation type techniques.

6. The aging nose

Aging is associated with changes in nasal aesthetics. These include downward rotation of the tip lobule, creating an acute columellar lobule angle, maxillary alveolar hypoplasia with resultant divergence of the medial crural feet and columellar shortening. The aesthetic result is a relatively longer nasal length, a droopy tip appearance and an apparently prominent dorsal hump (4).

7. Material and methods

7.1 Pretreatment considerations

Achieving satisfactory aesthetic outcomes relies on realistic expectations of properly selected patients in conjunction with precise execution of a selected technique that optimally addresses the deformity. During the initial interview, the patient's desires and goals should be carefully assessed in terms of realistic expectations of what can be accomplished. Medical history should be reviewed with focus on use of medication or supplements that might increase bleeding (e.g., nonsteroidal anti-inflammatory drugs, salicylate drugs, vitamin E, Omega-3, Ginseng, Ginko Biloba), allergies, history of cold sores, previous nasal operations or dermal filler treatments, and whether the patient is pregnant or lactating.

Before injection, the patient is counseled about the potential benefits against the inherent limitations of minimally invasive rhinosculpturing. Treatment course, possible adverse events, and the anticipated durability of treatment are reviewed. Following a full disclosure, informed consent is obtained and pretreatment photographs are taken in frontal, oblique, lateral and basal views.

7.2 Radiesse – the preferred injectable filler

Radiesse (Bioform Medical Inc, San Mateo, California) is an injectable filler material composed of synthetic CaHA microspheres (30%), suspended in an aqueous carrier gel (70%). CaHA is the primary constituent of bone and teeth and has been in use for more than 20 years in medicine (11,12).

Injectable CaHA is FDA approved for correction of moderate to severe facial wrinkles and folds and for restoration/correction of lipoatrophy in patients with HIV (13).

Following injection, the carrier gel is gradually absorbed and CaHA particles remain. Local histolocytic and fibroblastic response at the injection site result in neocollagenesis around the microspheres (14), thus contributing to the prolonged effects. Results achieved following injection remain almost unchanged until 12 months. After 12-18 months, the achieved volumes begin to diminish, though some results can be noted 24 months post-injection. The average longevity therefore could be considered to be 12-18 months (15-19). Longer duration of effect, up to 24 months, can be seen in some patients with a touch-up at one year of half the amount injected the first time (20).

CaHA was reported to generate longer lasting results and higher levels of patient satisfaction in 2 head to head studies with widely used HA fillers (21,22). Due to its composition and inherent biocompatibility, Radiesse is particularly suitable injectable material for augmentation of bony and cartilaginous contour deformities in the nasal area.

7.3 Pre-injection procedure

Before treatment, injection sites should be carefully marked by a washable marker with the patient in an upright position, and prepared with suitable antiseptic. Topical anesthesia using EMLA (lidocaine 2.5% and prilocane 2.5%) is applied for at least 15-20 minutes before injection. As regional infiltrative anesthesia frequently distorts surface landmarks, my personal preference is to premix 1cc of Radiesse with 0.3% lidocaine, a ratio equivalent to the widely used FDA-approved HA fillers. Radiesse is supplied in 1.5cc or 0.8 cc disposable syringes with Leur-lock fittings and should be injected with a 27-gauge 0.25 inch (6 mm) long needle.

7.4 Injection techniques

Radiesse should ordinarily be injected into the subdermal supraperiosteal plane in a retrograde fashion using a linear threading, fanning or cross-hatching technique, depending on the area being treated. The needle is placed at an angle of 30-45 degrees to the skin, and a subcutaneous space or track is created. Needle location is assessed with the index finger of the non-dominant hand to avoid visible nodules that might be created by superficial injection. Slow, continuous, even pressure applied to the syringe plunger whilst withdrawing the needle assures adequate control and helps to avoid product palpability. Frequent reassessment throughout the procedure is recommended when the patient is in the upright position, as the product is deposited incrementally. Overcorrection is to be avoided. As a practical rule, it is advisable to gradually achieve the final result over 2-3 sessions.

Systematic approach in rhinosculpturing is recommended starting with the nasal root and dorsum and proceeding to the supratip area, tip lobule and finally, the nasal base. Each injected area should address a specific deformity or aesthetic imperfection outlined during nasal examination and nasal aesthetic analysis. Important technical considerations and treatment goals will be discussed in relation to the above-mentioned anatomical regions:

Nasal root

Radiesse is injected into the supraperiosteal plane in the intended area using linear threading technique, starting in the midline. The index and thumb of the nondominant hand should be placed on either side of the nasal bones to prevent product migration. By doing so, the nasofrontal angle is increased (displaced cephalically), thus improving radix location in cases of low radix and the apparent short nose.

Nasal dorsum

Careful inspection of the light reflex from an upright standing position can reveal any irregularities in dorsal contour. Proper material deposition addresses dorsal contour irregularities, low radix, inverted V deformity, and improves the dorsal concavity of saddle nose deformity.

Nasal tip

The tip of the nose area is sensitive, so the injection point should be properly planned. It is recommended to start in the midline, slightly caudal to and between the tip-defining points, so a larger surface area can be approached using a single needle puncture. Injection depth is in the subcutaneous plane above the LLC. The index and thumb of the nondominant hand pinch the membranous caudal septum in order to alleviate pain and to stabilize the injected area. Next, the needle is advanced up to the supratip break point. (This point defines the cephalic limit of the nasal tip and is created by the difference between the projection of the tip-defining point and the height of the nasal dorsum.)

Injection while the needle is withdrawn can effectively correct a bifid tip and enhance tip projection. When continuing injection using the fanning technique, simulating an isosceles triangle, whose shanks point toward the medial portion of the lateral crura, pinched tip is improved and tip support is stabilized. This is especially the case when loss of tip support is due to excessive excision of the medial half of the lateral crus. By augmenting the inadequate skeletal support of the external valve, external valve incompetence can be improved.

Nasal base

Tip rotation, projection and support can be modified by augmentation. Injection of Radiesse into the central nasal base above the anterior nasal spine of the maxillary bone advances the premaxilla and opens the nasolabial angle, thus rotating the tip cephalically and improving a droopy tip. The needle is inserted at 45^0 to the upper lip toward the nasal spine and Radiesse is deposited 1 mm supraperiosteally while the index finger and thumb of the nondominant hand grasp the membranous septum cephalically. If further enhancement of tip support, projection and rotation is desired, augmentation material is placed between the medial crura toward the tip lobule, simulating columellar strut. By doing so, columellar show improves.

Functional nasal problems

Common causes of airway obstructions are internal and external valvular incompetence and inadvertent loss of tip support. Airway obstruction and loss of skeletal support require augmentation type procedures.

Spreader graft injection

With the aid of a head light, a double-hook or a nasal speculum is placed onto the nostrils. The alar rims are averted with the nondominant hand, thus exposing the internal nasal valve. Radiesse is injected into the submucoperichondrial and submucosal planes at the interface between the upper lateral cartilages and the dorsal cartilaginous septum using a 25-gauge 1.25 inch needle, in a retrograde linear threading technique. The injection serves as a spacer and opens the anterior septal angle, thereby increasing the cross-sectional area of the internal valve. This maneuver significantly increases the airflow into the nasal passages.

Alar batten graft injection

External valve incompetence requires structural support provided traditionally by placement of alar batten grafts. Once the site of collapse is identified during inspiration, the area is marked. The needle is threaded through the vestibule toward the supra-alar crease at the junction of the ULC and LLC, and injection is performed in a fanning technique. Alternatively, needle puncture is performed percutaneously toward the premarked area. Depth of injection reaches the subdermal and supra-perichondrial plane. Injection of alar batten reinforces the ala and nasal sidewall that had been prone to collapse with respiration. It should be noted that alar batten injection is difficult technically due to the tight skin envelope. Small doses, deposited over 2-3 sessions in an incremental fashion is recommended.

7.5 Post-injection consideration

Following injection, immediate molding and massage is advisable to smooth the surface and avoid irregularities. Injection site reactions such as redness and swelling are frequent and resolve spontaneously. Application of ice on to the injected areas helps to reduce tissue edema and ecchymosis. Patients are instructed to avoid the sun, tanning lights, sauna and intense facial treatment for at least 24 hours. Patient follow-up visits are typically scheduled 2 weeks post-injection. Micropore-like tapes are applied to the injected areas to diminish swelling. Refinement treatments are provided as needed.

8. Case presentations

8.1 Case presentation 1

Figure 4a. A 40-year-old female presented with inadequate tip projection and superior tip rotation ("porcine deformity") following rhinoplasty. A step-off deformity in the right nasal sidewall is presented secondary to overresection of the bony and cartilaginous roof. The lateral crus is deficient as well. The remaining cartilaginous rim appears knuckled owing to contractural healing forces acting on weakened cartilages (bossae) in a patient with thin skin. Physical examination revealed incompetence of the internal and external valves.

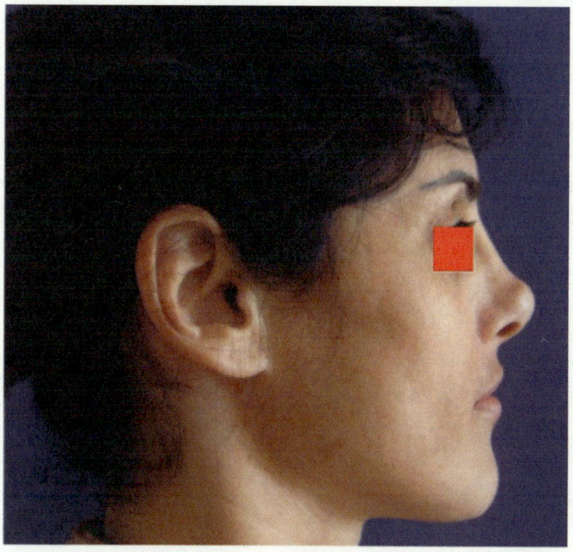

Fig. 4a. Preinjection lateral view demonstrating an inadequate tip projection, superior tip rotation, and step-off deformity in the right nasal side wall and bossae following prior rhinoplasty

Figure 4b. Post-injection photograph following spreader graft injection, and alar batten graft injection to support the internal and external valves, respectively. Radiesse™ was also injected to the nasal sidewall to smooth the step-off deformity and to the caudal dorsum at the supratip region to de-emphasize the overrotated tip (nasolabial angle was 104^0 before treatment and 92^0 following injection). Support of the skeletal deficient areas improved both form and function. The end result is an aesthetically pleasing nasal profile and well supported and projected tip.

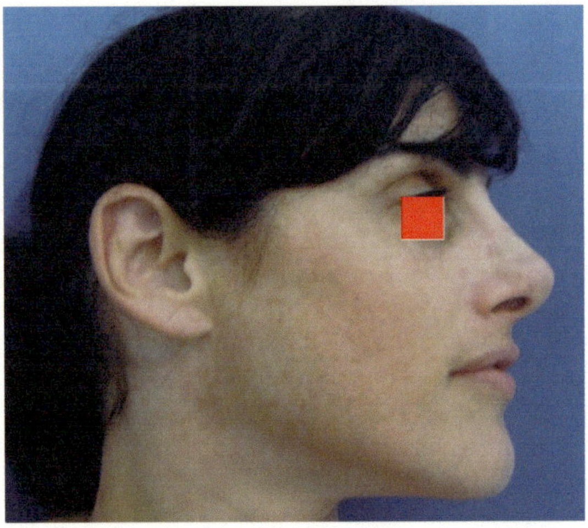

Fig. 4b. Postinjection lateral view showing improved nasal profile and well supported and projected tip

8.2 Case presentation 2

Figure 5a. Frontal view of a 47-year-old man with a history of 2 previous rhinoplastic surgeries and cartilage grafts (septal, conchal) placement during his revision rhinoplasty 5 years prior to presentation. Nasal examination revealed a deviated nasal bony base to right upper third, irregular nasal dorsum with slight saddle nose deformity, collapse of the left middle vault, collapse of both alar wings (left side greater than the right side), inadequate tip projection, asymmetric tip with deviation to the right, right side alar retraction and slightly retracted columella.

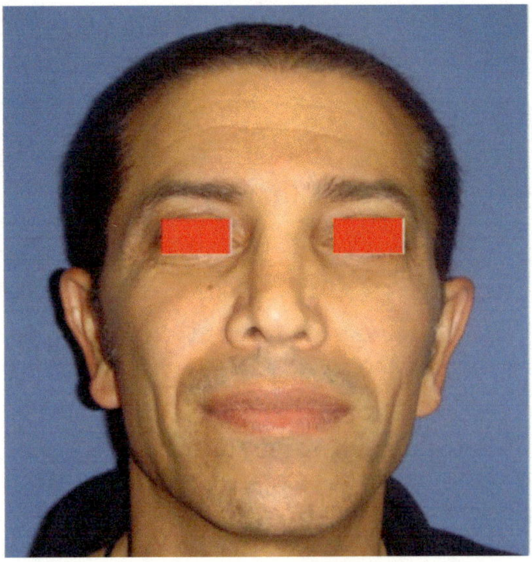

Fig. 5a. Preinjection frontal view demonstrating a deviated nasal bony base to the right, irregular nasal dorsum with slight saddle nose deformity, collapse of the left middle vault and alar wings and an asymmetric, inadequately projecting tip

Figure 5b. Frontal view following minimally invasive rhinosculpturing. Nasal sidewalls and dorsal augmentations were performed along with spreader grafts and alar batten graft injections. The unsightly right side bony irregularity was eliminated, the saddle deformity was corrected and dorsal contour was improved. Tip support was stabilized and symmetry was improved. Alar collapse was eliminated on the right side and improved on the left side (left alar collapse was eliminated in a subsequent session.) Spreader graft and alar batten graft injections enabled improved airflow due to the corresponding increase in the internal nasal valve angle and external valve area, respectively.

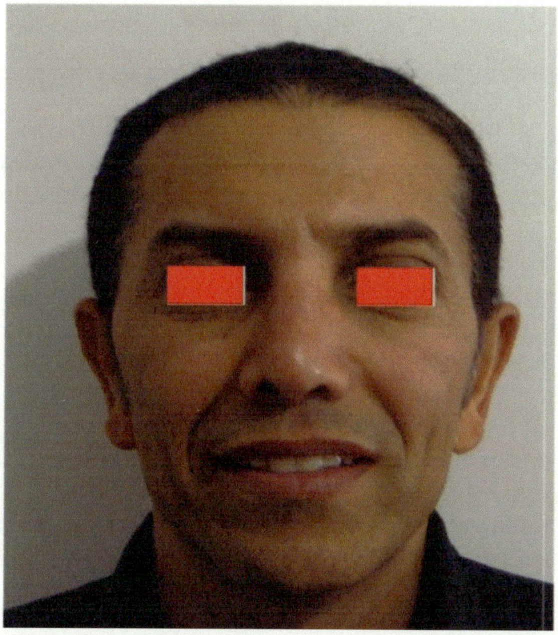

Fig. 5b. Frontal view following minimally invasive rhinosculpturing. Note the improved dorsal contour, enhanced nasal symmetry and smoothened skeletal irregularities

9. Discussion

During the last decade, minimally invasive rejuvenation procedures have gained widespread popularity and have become an indispensible component of today's modern cosmetic procedures. The diversity/blossoming of today's product options, recent innovations in injectable filler technology, and availability of fillers with documented safety profile, acceptable longevity, biocompatibility and low adverse problems pave the path to this paradigm shift. Moreover, minimally invasive facial procedures offer minimal downtime, less pain, no scars and a lower cost alternative compared to invasive procedures.

Rhinosculpturing using minimally invasive technique provides an attractive alternative to conventional rhinoplasty in selected cases. These include virgin noses necessitating augmentation type procedure for aesthetic refinement, correction of post-rhinoplasty contour defects, treating the aging and ethnic nose, and ameliorating/reversing selected functional nasal impairments. Nevertheless, conventional rhinoplasty remains a preeminent treatment in cases necessitating reduction type interventions, septal deformities, and nasal deformities otherwise not amenable to minimally invasive techniques.

As with any aesthetic procedure, the aesthetic outcome is the ultimate measure of proper selection and execution of a technique that is optimally tailored to the deformity addressed.

Inadequate nasal skeletal structure and support mandates the need for implant materials to improve both form and function. Augmentation materials can be broadly categorized as autografts, homografts, and alloplasts. An ideal augmentation material should approximate closely the shape, consistency and strength of the deficient nasal framework. It should be easily obtainable, capable of being shaped, biocompatible, resistant to extrusion or resorption by the body, and cost-effective. Myriad materials have been used over the years, each with its inherent advantages and liabilities (23).

Autologous cartilage grafts have become widely used as an effective autogenous supportive tissue. Sources include septal conchal and costal cartilage. If available, septal cartilage remains the cartilage of choice because of its rigidity, proximity, and straight contour. Septal grafts are commonly used as dorsal/radix grafts, spreader grafts, tip grafts, columellar struts and lateral crural and alar batten grafts. Despite their unsurpassed biocompatibility, disadvantages of cartilage grafts include limited supply, potential donor site morbidity, poorly predictable resorption rates and potential palpability, visibility or warping.

Injectable materials allow for non-invasive nasal augmentation and sculpture. Ideally, they should be non-toxic, non-allergic, biocompatible, easy to use, long lasting (yet, nonpermanent), inexpensive and reversible. They should demonstrate a high safety profile and produce a predictable result with minimal downtime.

Radiesse is a semi-solid, cohesive, completely biodegradable, deep subdermal implant. Its principle component is synthetic CaHA, the primary mineral constituent of bone and teeth. Results from *in vivo* and *in vitro* safety studies demonstrate that injectable CaHA is biocompatible, non-toxic, non-irritating and non-antigenic (24). Clinical, histologic and electron microscopic findings after *in vivo* injection have demonstrated dermal matrix integration in biopsy samples harvested from human volunteers (12). This CaHA injection provides scaffolding for collagen growth, thereby prolonging the duration of the effect. These histologic findings were accompanied by evidence of maintained clinical improvement (12). Biocompatibility studies on CaHA implants have all been characterized by minimal, if any, inflammatory response with no foreign body reaction or evidence of local systemic toxicity (11,12). Furthermore, there was neither ossification nor migration from the injection sites (20).

Two multicenter randomized trials comparing CaHA injections with the widely used HA fillers demonstrate that CaHA injections generate longer lasting results and higher levels of patient satisfaction (21,22). This might be explained by Radiesse's unique composition and by the higher elasticity and viscosity of Radiesse compared to the leading HA based dermal fillers (25).

Radiesse's chemical composition, physical properties and documented high safety profile render it valuable as the preferred injectable filler for augmentation type rhinosculpturing. Minimally invasive rhinosculpturing using Radiesse offers an attractive alternative to conventional rhinoplasty for patients who are actively hoping to avoid invasive surgery, and for those who are not candidates for surgery because of serious comorbidities. Patients wishing to appreciate the benefits of rhinosculpturing before a subsequent surgery and those who refuse revision surgery are likewise candidates for minimally invasive approach to rhinoplasty.

Selected functional nasal impairment can be ameliorated or even reversed via minimally invasive approach using Radiesse. Nyte (26) reported a spreader graft injection with Radiesse for a non-surgical solution in internal valve collapse in 23 patients. Alar batten graft injection with Radiesse can be used as a minimally invasive approach for external valve collapse. Radiesse might well serve as a viable alternative for other cartilage grafts such as dorsal cartilage graft, radix graft, tip grafts and columellar strut to contour structural nasal deficiencies. Cartilage graft injection using Radiesse spares donor sites, has minimal downtime, relatively longer term longevity, and is efficacious and cost-effective. Cartilage graft injection has low risk of extrusion, palpability or visibility.

Rhinosculpturing via minimally invasive approach should be considered as an alternative in cases mandating revision rhinoplasty where surgical expertise is of utmost importance. In those cases minimally invasive rhinosculpturing might spare the inevitable inherent difficulties posed on rhinoplasty in a previously operated nose.

In conclusion, Radiesse™ rhinosculpturing adds to the armamentarium of the rhinoplasty surgeon. It is an easy to perform procedure that might spare an operation and provides high patient satisfaction. Although much can be achieved by minimally invasive approach to rhinosculpturing, one must be cognizant of the fact that when selecting alternatives to address specific deformities, proper patient selection, detailed systematic analysis of the anatomical variables, artistic perception and precise execution are of paramount importance.

10. References

[1] Oneal RM, Beil RJ Jr, Schlensinger J. Surgical anatomy of the nose. Clin Plast Surg 1996;23(2):195-222.

[2] Powell N, Humphrey B. Proportions of the aesthetic face. New York: Thieme-Stratton; 1984.

[3] Tardy ME, Becker DG, Weingerg MS. Illusion in rhinoplasty. Facial Plast Surg 1995;11:117-138.

[4] Rohrich RJ, Hollier JR LH, Janis JE, Kim J. Rhinoplasty with advancing age. Plast Reconstr Surg 2003;114(7):1936-1944.

[5] Larrabee WFJr. Facial beauty. myth or reality. Arch Otolaryngol Head Neck Surg 1997;123:571-2

[6] American Society for Aesthetic Plastic Surgery. 1997-2010 Cosmetic Surgery National Data Bank Statistics. http://www.surgery.org. Accessed October,10 2010.

[7] Petroff MA, McCollough EG, Hom D, Anderson JR. Nasal tip projection: quantitative changes following rhinoplasty. Arch Otolaryngol Head Neck Surg 1991;117:783-8.

[8] Ricketts RM. Divine proportion in facial esthetics. Clin Plast Surg 1982:9:401-22.

[9] Constantian MB. Practical nasal aesthetics. In: Habal M, ed. Advances in Plastic and Reconstructive Surgery. St Louis, Mosby-Year Book, 1991:85-107.

[10] Becker DG, Becker SS. Reducing complications in rhinoplasty. Otolaryngol Clin North Am 2006;39:475-92.

[11] Havlik RJ; PSEF DATA Committee. Hydroxylapatite. Plast Reconstr Surg 2002;15:1176-9.

[12] Hobar PC, Pantaloni M, Byrd MS. Porous hydroxyapatite granules for alloplastic enhancement of the facial region. Clin Plast Surg 2000;27:557-69.

[13] Radiesse [package insert], San Mateo, CA: Bioform Medical Inc., 2009.

[14] Marmur ES, Phelps R, Goldberg D, Marmur et al. (2004) Clinical, histologic and electron microscopic findings after injection of a calcium hydroxylapatite filler. J Cosmet Laser Ther. 2004 Dec;6(4):223-6.

[15] Tzikas TL. Evaluation of Radiesse FN: A new soft tissue filler. Dermatol Surg 2004;30:764-8.

[16] Kanchwala SL, Holloway L, Bucky LP. Reliable soft tissue augmentation: a clinical comparison of injectable soft-tissue fillers for facial-volume augmentation. Ann Plast Surg 2005;55:30-5.

[17] Jacovella PF. Calcium hydroxylapatite facial filler (Radiesse): indications, technique, and results. Clin Plast Surg 2006;33:511-23.

[18] Jansen DA, Graivier MH. Evaluation of calcium hydroxylapatite-based implant (Radiesse) for facial soft tissue augmentation. Plast Reconstr Surg 2006 Sep;118(3 Suppl):22S-30S, discussion 31S-33S.

[19] Silvers SL, Eviatar JA, Echavez MI, Pappas AL. Prospective, open-label, 18-month trial of calcium hydroxylapatite (Radiesse) for facial soft-tissue augmentation in patients with human immunodeficiency virus-associated lipoatrophy: one-year durability. Plast Reconstr Surg 2006 Sep;118(3 Suppl):34S-45S.

[20] Feldmerman LI. Radiesse for facial rejuvenation. Cosmet Dermatol 2005;18:823-6.

[21] Moers Carpi MM, Tufet JO. Calcium hydroxylapatite versus nonanimal stabilized hyaluronic acid for the correction of nasolabial folds: a 12-month, multicenter, prospective, randomized, controlled, split-face trial. Dermatol Surg 2008 Feb;34(2):210-5.

[22] Moers-Carpi M, Vogt S, Santos BM, Planas J, Vallve SR, Howell DJ. A multicenter, randomized trial comparing calcium hydroxylapatite to two hyaluronic acids for treatment of nasolabial folds. Dermatol Surg. 2007;33 Suppl 2:S144-51.

[23] Lovice DB, Mingrone MD, Toriumi DH. Grafts and implants in rhinoplasty and nasal reconstruction. Otolaryngol Clin North Am 1999;32(1):113-41.

[24] Hubbard WH. Bioform implants. Biocompatibility. Franksville, Wis: Bioform, Inc., 2003.

[25] BioForm Medical Inc., 2009, data on file.

[26] Nyte CP. Spreader graft injection with calcium hydroxylapatite: a nonsurgical technique for internal valve collapse. Laryngoscope 2006:116:1291-2

Part 6

Complications

10

Mucous Cysts as a Complication of Rhinoplasty

Aris Ntomouchtsis[1], Nikos Kechagias[1], Persefoni Xirou[2], Georgios Christos Balis[2], Katerina Xinou[3] and Konstantinos Vahtsevanos[1]
[1]*Department of Oral and Maxillofacial Surgery, Theagenion Cancer Hospital, Thessaloniki*
[2]*Department of Histopathology, Theagenion Cancer Hospital, Thessaloniki*
[3]*Department of Radiology, Theagenion Cancer Hospital, Thessaloniki*
Greece

1. Introduction

Aesthetic and reconstructive surgery of the nose remains the most challenging and difficult of all head and neck plastic surgical operations. (Tardy, 1995) Rhinoplasty is considered as a highly demanding procedure. The nose is the most prominent part of the face and derogations may be less appropriate than deviations.

Complications can refer either to the skeletal framework or to the soft-tissue regions and they can be divided into functional and aesthetical. According to the time of presentation they can be intraoperative or postoperative early or late complications.

Implantation cysts and deforming masses are infrequent and very rare, but avoidable complications of rhinoplasty. Displacement of fragments of epithelium may result in subcutaneous graft entrapment and subsequent encystation. Epidermoid cysts or mucous cysts may be developed, depending on the type of epithelium trapped. They must be addressed with a thorough evaluation of the extent of the lesion to choose the most appropriate procedure for removal. Knowledge of the various capabilities and presentations of postrhinoplasty cysts, will better equip surgeons for a successful outcome. Although a mucous cyst is a benign lesion, it is considered to be a serious complication of rhinoplasty. Mucous cysts are presented in many locations and ages, with a wide range of concurrent symptoms. Most of them are appeared several months or years after rhinoplasty.

Complete resection of the mucous cyst is the gold standard of treatment. Identification of involved structures will ensure appropriate procedure selection. Almost all the cases reported in the literature have been described as solitary lesions which were successfully eradicated following a single surgical procedure.

There was only one paper reported a case of a patient who had presented two mucous cysts,the first one two months postoperatively and the second one five months after surgical extirpation (Mouly, 1970), and only two authors reported recurrence after surgical intervention. (Zijlker and Vuyk, 1993; Ntomouchtsis et.al. 2010) Regarding the high number of rhinoplasty procedures performed worldwide every year, the number of the 30 published cases is on the contrary very low. These observations make it possible that specific local conditions must exist before a mucous cyst may be expected to develop and one important factor is likely to be the size of the displaced epithelial fragment. There is also exists the possibility that all occurred complications have not been presented yet.

It is interesting that there have been two reports of respiratory implantation cysts of the mandible following combined rhinoplasty and genioplasty, where the chin augmentation is achieved using osteocartilagenous grafts harvested from the nasal dorsum. (Anastassov and Lee, 1999; Imholte and Schwartz, 2001)
A thorough evaluation of the extent of the lesion is the best way for the surgeon to choose the most appropriate procedure for removal.

2. Clinical signs and differential diagnosis

Patients normally complain about a gradually swelling mass in the operation field or in its proximity. They may also feel continuous pressure over the lesion. Cysts may be featured as circular, mobile and non tender mass when they are palpated. Otherwise it can be an immobile, painless, soft smooth subcutaneous mass fixed to the skin and to the deep planes. The overlying skin tends to be more vascular than the closest region.
Functional and aesthetic problems could be caused by the lesion, such as remarkable asymmetry of the tip and the nostrils, persistent nasal obstruction and increased snoring, impaired nasal breathing and swelling, deviation of the septum and saddle nose deformity. Symptoms and signs of inflammation, like infection and abscess formation, can accompany the mass. (Zijlker and Vuyk, 1993; Flaherty et al., 1996; Kotzur and Gubisch, 1997; Bracaglia et al.,2005; Tastan et al.,2010 It has been reported that antibiotics have managed to halt the enlargement but can not always achieve resolution of the cysts. (Shulman and Westreich, 1983; Dini, 2001)
The main differential diagnosis of mucous cyst must also includes other entities beyond infections, such as lipogranulomas/ paraffinomas, which are thought to represent foreign body reactions to displaced lipid ointment from nasal packings through intranasal incisions. (Gryskiewicz, 2001) Other various benign tumor-like nasal lesions must be taken under consideration, such as epidermoid inclusion cysts, tumefective cartilage proliferation, osteomas, lipomas, pleomorphic salivary adenomas, granulomatous diseases. Congenital midline nasal masses including, gliomas, encephaloceles, and nasal dermoid sinus cysts are reported to occur. Lesions such as inverting papillomas, juvenile nasopharyngeal angiofibroma, ethesioneuroblastoma and even frontal sinus mucoceles must be excluded. (Baarsma , 1980; Hacker and Freeman , 1994; Romo T 3rd et al. 1999) It could be harmful to misdiagnose malignant neoplastic lesions that can involve the nasal region such as squamous cell carcinoma, malignant melanoma, adenocarcinoma, sarcoma, and lymphoma.
Clinical examination, nasal endoscopy, imaging studies and finally cytology or/and histological analysis after biopsy will define the possible diagnosis.
The sites of mucous cyst occurrence can vary. The majority of these these cysts occur over the nasal bone along the line of nasal osteotomy, with the nasal dorsum being the most affected site. **Table 1.** In few cases, rare locations have been described, including paranasally along the maxillary osteotomy, (Karapantzos et.al., 1999; Raine et.al., 2003), the lateral wall, the tip of the nose, the alar, the inner canthus, the radix nasi, and even the glabellar region. (Mouly, 1970; Rettinger and Zenkel, 1997; Bracaglia et al. 2005; Riedel et.al. 2007; Pausch et al. 2010; Ntomouchtsis et al. 2010; Dionyssopoulos et al. 2010)

3. Radiologic findings

The list of differential diagnoses ranges from postoperative nasal lesions, various other benign, congenital, infectious or neoplastic processes unrelated to surgery.

A/A	Author	Year	Sex/Age	Location	Duration	Rhinoplasty
1	McGregor	1958	N.A.	Dorsum	5 days	Direct open
2	Mouly	1970	F/N.A.	Canthus inner bilateral	2m & 5m	Direct open
3	Senechal	1981	M/31	Radix	10y	Direct open
4	» »	» »	F/44	Paranasal	8y	Direct open
5	Shulman	1983	F/32	Dorsum/Tip	2m	closed
6	Lawson	1983	M/28	Dorsum	Several m	Direct open
7	Harley	1990	F/27	Dorsum	6y	closed
8	» »	» »	M/22	Dorsum	10m	closed
9	Toriumi	1990	N.A	N.A	N.A	N.A
10	Zijlker	1993	F/31	Dorsum	1y	open
11	Flaherty	1996	F/24	Dorsum	5y	closed
12	Kotzur	1997	M/45	Dorsum	6y	Direct open
13	» »	» »	M/23	Dorsum	4y	closed
14	» »	» »	M/24	Dorsum	2y	closed
15	Rettinger	1997	M/N.A	Alar lateral	1y	Direct open
16	Karapantzos	1999	M/25	Paranasal	3m	Direct open
17	Romo	1999	M/33	Dorsum	2y	Direct open
18	Tan Ergin	2000	M/47	Dorsum	6m	Direct open
19	Dini	2001	M/29	Dorsum	3m	Direct open
20	Raine	2003	F/58	Paranasal	20y	close
21	Liu	2003	M/33	Dorsum	7y	Direct open
22	Bracaglia	2005	F/30	Lateral Wall	2m	Endoscopic
23	» »	» »	F/38	Radix	1y	Endoscopic
24	Riedel	2007	F/34	Lateral Wall	6m	close
25	Pausch	2010	F/17	Dorsum	14m	open
26	» »	» »	F/19	Alar lateral	1y	open
27	Struijs	2010	M/64	Dorsum	40y	open
28	Tastan	2010	F/25	Tip	1y	open
29	Dionyssopoulos	2010	F/26	Glabella	22m	Direct open
30	» »	» »	F/20	Canthus inner	6 m	open
31	Ntomouchtsis	2010	F/29	Glabella	15m	Direct open

Table 1. Table of all published cases in the English literature

Preoperative assessment with computed tomography and/or magnetic resonance imaging can help narrow the differential diagnosis by evaluating the nature of contents within the

mass and the possibility of bony or intracranial involvement. (Leong and Sharp, 2009) CT assesses for any bony involvement, while MRI gives better definition of soft tissues and is likely the best method for detecting intracranial masses. (Barkovich et al., 1991)
A CT scan or magnetic resonance imaging is needed to determine the extent of the lesion and thus the best surgical approach. Magnetic resonance imaging gives a more detailed image and has fewer false-negatives and fewer false-positives than CT. (Zerris et al., 2002)
Only 3 of the 31 reported cases have described the radiological (CT or MR) features of postrhinoplasty mucous cysts. (Raine et al., 2003; Leong and Sharp, 2009; Ntomouchtsis et al., 2010)

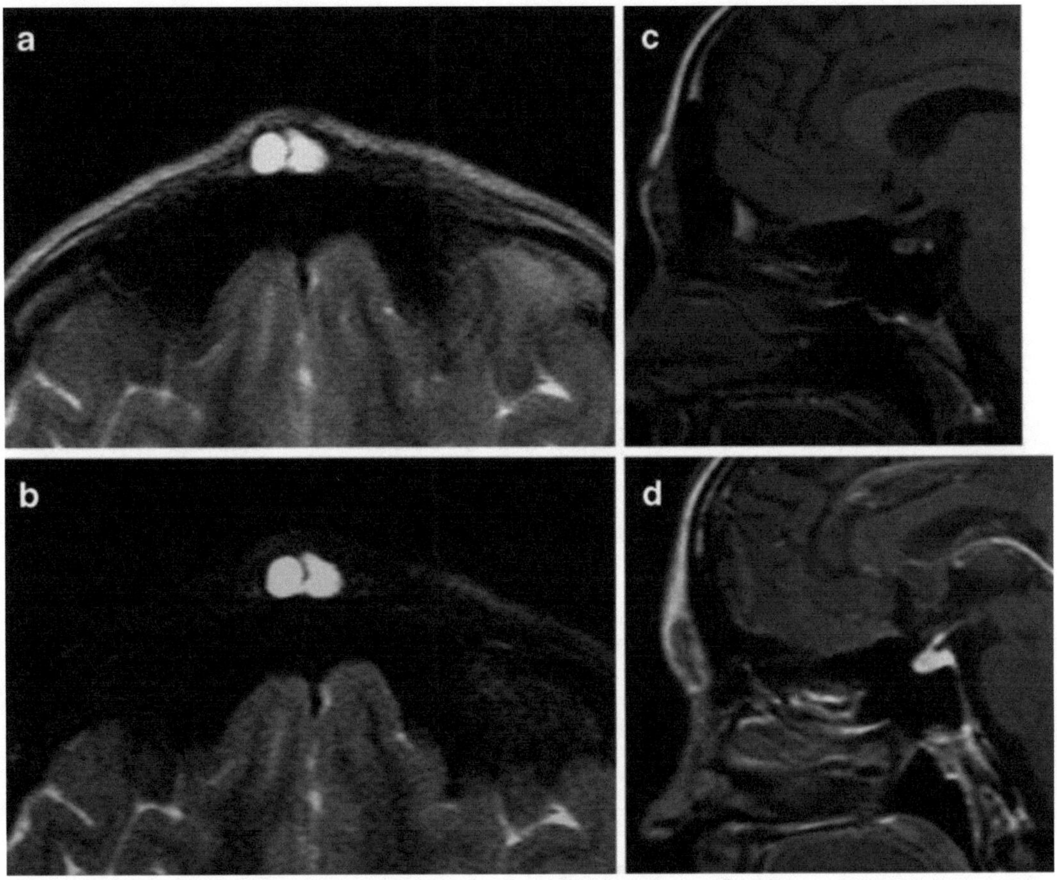

Fig. 1. a–d Brain MRI showing an oval-shaped subcutaneous cystic lesion in the midline, in front of the frontal sinuses. The lesion shows homogeneously high signal intensity in axial T2 (a) and STIR images (b), low signal intensity in sagittal T1-weighted image (c), and peripheral enhancement in sagittal T1-weighted image after gadolinium injection (d)

A CT scan or magnetic resonance imaging is needed to determine the extent of the lesion and thus the best surgical approach. Magnetic resonance imaging gives a more detailed image and has less false-negatives and less false-positives than CT. (Zerris et al., 2002) CT assess for any intracranial connection. MRI which gives better definition of soft tissues is likely the best method for detecting intracranial masses. (Barkovich et al., 1991)

Mucous cysts usually appear as well-defined, homogenous, non-enhancing or peripherally enhancing lesions with no bony destruction and without any intracranial communication. The content of these cysts is mostly hypointense in CT, and shows low to intermediate signal in T1-weighted and high signal in T2-weighted images in MR. (Koeller et al., 1999; Leong and Sharp, 2009; Ntomouchtsis et al., 2010) Unfortunately, these findings are not specific because they can be encountered also in foreign body inclusion cysts (Pausch et al., 2010), epidermoid cysts and sebaceous cysts. Raine et al described a case of a mucous cyst, which appeared as a well-defined hypointense soft tissue mass in CT with no bony elements, findings more consistent with a fibrous or granulomatous lesion. (Raine et al., 2003)
The differential diagnosis of mucous cysts from paraffinomas, dermoid cysts and lipomas is easier, because the latter are fat-containing hypointense lesions in CT, usually showing high signal in T1- and T2-weighted images in MR. (Koeller et al., 1999; Liu et al., 2003)
Therefore, CT and MR imaging is helpful in the preoperative evaluation of a post-rhinoplasty lesion, because it can demonstrate the benign nature and the cystic content of the mass, excluding other benign non-enhancing lesions (granuloma, sebaceous cyst, dermoid cyst, lipoma), solid enhancing lesions (traumatic aneurysm, hemangioma, neurofibroma, lymphoma, basal cell carcinoma, metastasis) or lesions that cover underlying calvarial masses (eosinophilic granuloma, meningioma, metastasis). Color Doppler ultrasonography can also be used in differential diagnostic problems of cystic lesions as an alternative of MRI. (Riedel et al., 2007) If any concern exists as to the possible diagnosis, a preoperative biopsy should be considered.

4. Surgery

Surgical eradication remains the appropriate treatment for mucous cysts of the nose. Complete resection avoiding rupture is curative. The surgical procedure is dependent on the location and extent of the lesion and on patient age. The reconstruction of the intraoperatively resulting defect is a challenging problem, which has to be solved, mainly from a aesthetic point of view.
Many surgical approaches have been described and successfully attempted as presented in the literature. Endonasal intercartilagineous and intracartilagineous incisions, although they offer limited exposure, they have been used successfully for mucous cysts involving the tip and supratip regions. (Flaherty et al., 1996; Kotzur and Gubisch, 1997; Shulman and Westreich, 1983; ; Dionyssopoulos et al. 2010) Extracolumellar incision is used for an open rhinoplasty technique. It gives excellent exposure for complete extirpation of the lesion and reconstruction of the defect and leaves inconspicuous scars in the long run. Incision through the overlying skin of the lesion permits direct and excellent exposure but must be considered as a third option due to visible scars are leaved.
The direct percutaneous approach, even when a geometrically broken line incision is used, may result in a visible scar. There has even been an endoscopic approach proposed. (Bracaglia et al., 2005)
The open approach through the existing scars should be preferred for revision of rhinoplasty in cleft lip patients. (Pausch et al., 2010)
Dorsal nasal cysts formation is prevented by extremely meticulous removement of all debris from the operative site by suction and submucosal separation of the upper lateral cartilages. There are two ways of dealing with the upper lateral cartilages where they are attached to the septum. The mucosa can either be detached and left intact or released by a transmucosal

incision by using "junction tunnels", which preserve the mucosa. The mucoperichondrium and mucoperiosteum are elevated bilaterally at the junction of the septum with the nasal wall. The upper lateral cartilage is released by preserving the mucosal integrity through submucosal dissection. Entrapment of mucosa and formation of nasal cysts should be prevented by maintaining intact the mucosal integrity under osteotomy or cartilage incision sites. (Johnson and Anderson, 1977; Ress, 1980) Creation of dead space is declined by trying to avoid undermining osteotomy sites.
Irrigation at the end of the procedure can provide additional clearing of remnants from the surgical field. Careful removal of all mucosal fragments from the osteotomy sites at the time of primary surgery is mandatory and can by preventative.
Complete surgical extirpation of cysts may lead to disfigurement of the nasal framework.
Direct reconstruction of the defect sets the goal of surgical treatment of this rare condition. Cartilaginous grafts (e.g., rib or concha grafts) are recommended for reconstruction of the nasal frame in such cases.

5. Intraoperative findings

On exploration the cystic mass could appear as a distinct capsule with no direct connection between it and the nasal mucosa, as it has been reported in the majority of the published cases. (Harley and Erdman, 1990; Romo T 3rd et al., 1999) On the other hand the cyst could be found either tightly attached to the surrounding tissues, or adherent to the overlying skin, or in connection with the underlying cartilaginous and bony nasal structures, or even attached to previously used autogenous grafts. (Kotzur and Gubisch, 1997; Tan Ergin and Akkuzu , 2000; Pausch et al., 2010)
The underlying nasal bone or cartilage in the area of the lesion can be depressed with an impression deformity, or eroded or even resorbed. [21,30,31] (Harley and Erdman, 1990; Tan Ergin and Akkuzu , 2000; Pausch et al., 2010)
During the operation the lesion can be removed removed either intact or perforated.If the latter happens, clear fluid or partly fatty fluid or mucous fluid or even thick white-yellowish liquid usually is yielded from the cystic wall. (Flaherty et al., 1996; Kotzur and Gubisch, 1997; Romo T 3rd et al., 1999)
Dead space or deformity of bone or cartilage could be created,in the operation field, after complete cyst removal. which has to be managed through careful suturing in layers and to be repaired, usually by using autogenous graft.

6. Histopathology

Macroscopically a mucous cyst appears as an oval shaped,soft smooth walled cyst, located subcutaneously, easily separated from its surrounding structures and filled with mucinous material. Microscopically the cyst wall is lined by ciliated columnar respiratory type epithelium with dispersed goblet cells. (Ntomouchtsis et al., 2010)
Due to the fact that diagnosis is based primarily on microscopic findings, particularly the lining of the cysts, similar cutaneous cystic formations can enter in the differential diagnosis. Cutaneous ciliated cysts show numerous papillary projections lined by a simple cuboidal or columnar ciliated epithelium, while mucin-secreting cells are absent. These cysts can be found on the lower extremities (females) or on the back (males) and measure several centimeters in diameter. (Elder et al., 2010)

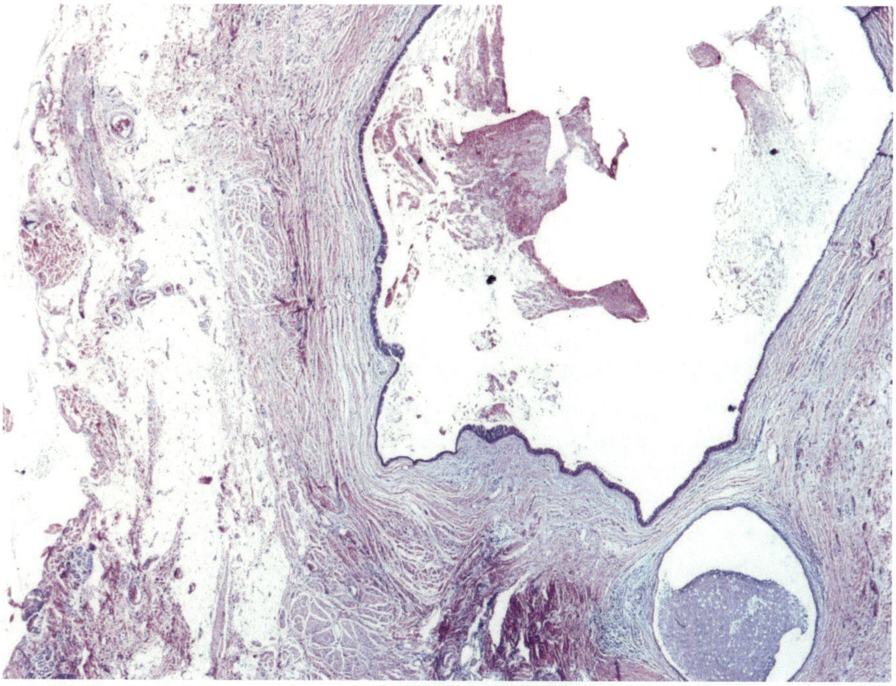

Fig. 2. Cyst filled with mucinous material (H-E ×20)

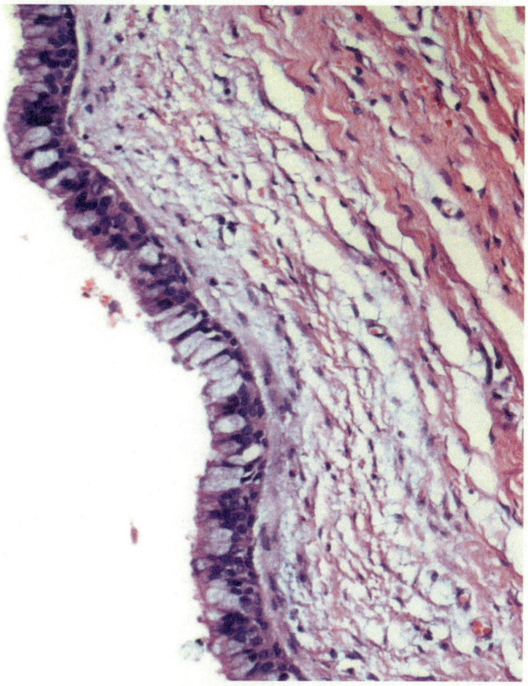

Fig. 3. The cyst wall is lined by ciliated columnar respiratory type epithelium with dispersed goblet cells (H-E ×200)

Bronchogenic cysts are lined by a mucosa consisting of ciliated pseudostratified columnar epithelium, while goblet cells may be interspersed. The wall frequently contains smooth muscle and mucous glands. Thyroglossal duct cysts differ from bronchogenic cysts in that they do not contain smooth muscle and they frequently contain thyroid follicles. Bronchogenic cysts are most commonly seen on the suprasternal notch and rarely on the anterior aspect of the neck or on the chin. Thyroglossal duct cysts are clinically indistinguishable from bronchogenic cysts, except that they are usually located on the anterior aspect of the neck. (Elder et al., 2010)

Apocrine hidrocystoma is a multi-loculated cystic lesion with occasional papillary projections. The inner surface of the cyst and the papillary projections are lined by a row of columnar secretory cells of variable height showing decapitation secretion indicative of apocrine secretion. Peripheral to the layer of secretory cells are elongated myoepithelial cells, their long axes running parallel to the cyst wall. Apocrine hidrocystoma occurs usually as a solitary, translucent cystic nodule on the face and occasionally on the ears, scalp, chest, shoulders, or vulva. Multiple apocrine hidrocystomas are rarely encountered. Frequently, the lesion has a blue hue, while the diameter ranges from 1 to 20 mm. (Elder et al., 2010)

Eccrine hidrocystoma shows a single cystic cavity, while the cyst wall usually shows two layers of small, cuboidal epithelial cells. In some areas, only a single layer of flattened epithelial cells can be seen, their flattened nuclei extending parallel to the cyst wall. Small papillary projections extending into the cavity of the cyst are observed rarely. Eccrine secretory tubules and ducts are often located below the cyst and in close approximation to it, and, on serial sections, one may find an eccrine duct leading into the cyst from below. However, no connection can be found between the cyst and the epidermis. In this condition, usually one lesion -- but occasionally several, and rarely numerous lesions -- are present on the face. As in apocrine hidrocystoma, the lesion consists of a small, translucent, cystic nodule 1 to 3 mm in diameter that often has a bluish hue. (Elder et al., 2010)

Cutaneous metaplastic synovial cysts show villous-like projections and a lining that resembles hyperplastic synovium (not epithelium). This type of cysts is rare and presents months or years after a surgery as solitary tender subcutaneous nodule. The cause of formation of cutaneous metaplastic synovial cysts remains unclear, but previous trauma usually precedes their onset. Taking in consideration this entity is significant, since a recent publication reports a case of cutaneous metaplastic synovial cyst on a patient's face after receiving hyaluronic acid filler injections. (Inchingolo et al., 2010)

Foreign body inclusion cysts, even though called cysts inappropriately, microscopically they represent granulomatous reaction to bone or cartilage fragments following rhinoplasty. [34] (Chang and Jin, 2008)

Follicular cysts (epidermal, trichilemmal, dermoid, etc) can be often found on the face, regardless of any previous intervention, but can easily be excluded from the diagnosis since they are lined by stratified squamous epithelium resembling epidermis and filled with keratinous material. Even though we should be aware of this type of cysts since there have been reports of post rhinoplasty epidermal cysts. (Grocutt and Fatah, 1989; Tastan et al., 2010)

All of the aforementioned cysts show similar clinical or pathological findings with the cutaneous mucous cysts, but a careful histological examination can spot the differences and exclude them from the diagnosis.

In conclusion, histological examination of all cysts that present on the face after an intervention is of paramount importance, not only to exclude malignancy, but also to narrow down the list of differential diagnoses.

7. Theories of creation

The aetiology of this lesion remains unknown and controversial. Different theories of creation exist. The first hypothesis assumes the herniation of nasal mucosa in the direct postoperative period, for example after a patient blew his or her nose. (McGregor et al., 1958) The herniation or subsequent growth of nasal mucosa can take place through the infracture sites or incisions, although no reported cases mentioned any connection of a cyst to the normal mucous layer of the nose. (Mouly, 1970; Harley and Erdman, 1990)

The most reasonable explanation is the proliferation of ectopic or displaced mucous membranes, followed by improper clearing of mucous epithelial remnants and bony or cartilage parts. This seeding of mucous tissue and remnants attached to bone or cartilage either in situ or as a part of an autogenous graft seems to be the main reason for which the mucous grafts grow and proliferate in their ectopic position (Shulman and Westreich, 1983; Harley and Erdman, 1990; Kotzur and Gubisch, 1997; Dini et al., 2001)

Another aspect that has to be emphasized is that in some of the described cases in the literature, the location of appearance does not coincide with the osteotomy lines or even with the intervention field of a rhinoplasty. This could be explained by poor surgical technique during a close rhinoplasty, which can lead to extreme surgical trauma, violation of the intranasal mucosal lining and subsequent encystation of nasal mucosal epithelium, displaced at the time of surgery. (Zijlker and Vuyk, 1993; Dini et al., 2001; Ntomouchtsis et al., 2010) This explains the different locations described in the literature, and the absence of connections with the internal nasal lining that is observed and described during surgical eradication.

On the other hand, the reappearance of a cyst can also be attributed to a faulty surgical technique. (Ntomouchtsis et al., 2010) It is also hypothesized that cysts may develop by occlusion of sebaceous glands because of scar tissue formation. (Rettinger and Zenkel, 1997)

In cleft lip nose rhinoplasty, however, cystic masses of the nose might have other origins, so congenital malformations or remnants of the nasolacrimal duct have also been described. Mucous cysts of the nose are not specific complications of cleft nose surgery, although they have been observed in this specific patients group. (Aikawa et al., 2008; Pausch et al., 2010)

8. Prevention

In order to prevent iatrogenic cyst formation it is important to use an appropriate surgical technique. The manoeuvres must be executed carefully with respect to the soft and hard tissues of the operation field. The need for atraumatic and careful tissue dissection has been emphasized by virtually all authors who have described postrhinoplasty mucous cysts.

By preserving the mucosal integrity and using sharp instruments one can hope to avoid the involuntary dispersion of tissues into other layers while dissecting. The mucosal lining must be kept intact during the rhinoplasty, or in any case of disruption a meticulously restoration is mandatory. Mucosal lining can be preserved when subperichondrial and subperiostal tunnels are being established over the septum and under the nasal dorsum before any surgical alterations will be made to the structures. (Zijlker and Vuyk, 1993) Completing of all osteotomies is also important for maintaining mucosal integrity during intranasal osteotomy and to decrease the chance of cyst formation. The osteotomy sites must be placed properly, and performed with adequate water injection and hydrodissection. The mucosa around the lateral osteotomy site should be elevated, to prevent entrapment. For security the osteotomy sites should be thoroughly inspected at the completion of the procedure. (Liu and Kridel, 2003).

On the other hand many surgeons prefer not to elevate tunnels, as this additional stripping and dissection of periosteum decreases the structural support of the nasal framework after osteotomies are complete. They report better stability and more predictable outcomes with external perforated osteotomy, by using a small osteotome (2-4 mm) that simultaneously minimize disruption of periosteal surfaces, stabilize medial movement, reduce lateral wall collapse and decreases dead space. (Goldfarb et al., 1993; Rohrich et al., 2001; Rohrich et al., 2003) It as experimentally been shown that this technique decreases soft-tissue disruption or displacement compared to continuous osteotomies. (Byrne et al., 2003) It must also be emphasized that none of the reported postrhinoplasty cysts are connected to this surgical technique.

Meticulous removal of all bony, cartilaginous and mucous remnants is essential. It is essential that if osteocartilagenous grafts are used harvested from the nasal frame they must be prepared by removing the respiratory epithelium prior to implantation. (Raine et al., 2003) Irrigation at the end of the procedure can be an additional measure to clear the surgical field of remnants. (Gryskiewicz, 2001) The created dead space must be closed in layers. Intranasal incisions should be closed properly. Rhinoplasty is a very demanding procedure. In complicated cases, especially in revision surgery, the risk of complications is higher when performed by inexperienced surgeons. The best prevention of mucous cysts occurring after rhinoplasty is not only meticulous elimination of all bony, cartilage, and epithelial tissues and mucous parts, but also, and even more important, emphasis on a most atraumatic and careful operation. (Kotzur and Gubisch, 1997) The key to a good outcome is localizing the lesion and selecting the most appropriate procedure.

9. Conclusion

Relative to the high number of rhinoplasty procedures performed each year worldwide, the number of the 31 presented published cases is on the contrary very low. (Senechal et al., 1981; Lawsonet al., 1983; Toriumi and Johnson, 1990; Struijs and Bauwens, 2010) The only data reported regarding the frequency of postrhinoplasty mucous cysts are from two case reports, where there are count 1/6000 and 3/5000, a percentage of 0.02 and 0.06 respectively. (Kotzur and Gubisch, 1997; Dini et al., 2001) Otherwise there is a large number of unreported cases or the postrhinoplasty cyst is a really rare condition. (Karapantzos et al., 1999)

It is possible that intraoperative tissue dispersion would occur in large number of cases, but does not lead automatically to the development of cysts. Although the physiopathology is uncertain, it seems that entrapped fragments of epithelial tissue are proliferated, if specific local conditions are created. It remains unclear what factors influence the final formation in these rare cases.

10. References

Aikawa T, Iida S, Fukuda Y, Nakano Y, Ota Y, Takao K, Kogo M. Nasolabial cyst in a patient with cleft lip and palate. Int J Oral Maxillofac Surg. 2008;37:874–876.

Anastassov GE, Lee H. Respiratory mucocele formation after augmentation genioplasty with nasal osteocartilagenous graft. J Oral Maxillofac Surg 1999;57:1263–5.

Baarsma EA. The median nasal sinus and dermoid cyst. Arch Otorhinolaryngol 1980;226:107- 13.

Barkovich J, Vandermarck P, Edwards M, Cogen PH. Congenital nasal masses: CT and MR imaging features in 16 cases. A J Neuroradiol 1991;12,105-116

Bracaglia R, Fortunato R,Gentileschi S Endoscopic excision for postrhinoplasty mucous cyst of the nose. Br J Plast Surg. 2005 Mar;58(2):271-4.

Byrne PJ, Walsh WE, Hilger PA. The use of "inside-out" lateral osteotomies to improve outcome in rhinoplasty. Arch Facial Plast Surg. 2003 May-Jun;5(3):251-5.

Chang DY, Jin HR. (2008). Foreign Body Inclusion Cyst of the Nasal Radix after Augmentation Rhinoplasty. J Korean Med Sci. 23, 6, pp. 1109-12.

Dini M, Innocenti A, Agostini V. Postrhinoplasty mucous cyst of the nose. Plast Reconstr Surg. 2001;107:885- 886.

Dionyssopoulos A, Nikolis A, Papaconstantino A,Kaka P, Miliaras D,Keke Gs, Mucous Cysts of the Nose: A Postrhinoplasty Complication? A Long-Term Follow-UpAnn Plas Surg 2010; 64(4),381-4

Elder DE, Elenitsas R, Johnson BL Jr., Murphy GF, Xu X (2010). Lever's Histopathology of the Skin, Chapters 29-30

Goldfarb M, Gallups JM, Gerwin J.M. Perforating osteotomies in rhinoplasty. *Arch. Otolaryngol. Head Neck Surg.* 119: 624, 1993.

Flaherty G, Pestalardo CM, Itturalde JG et al (1996) Mucous cyst: postrhinoplasty complications. Aesthetic Plast Surg 20:29–31

Grocutt M, Fatah MF. (1989). Recurrent multiple epidermoid inclusion cysts following rhinoplasty--an unusual complication. J Laryngol Otol.103, 12, pp. 1214-6.

Gryskiewicz JM. Paraffinoma or postrhinoplasty mucous cyst of the nose: which is it? Plast Reconstr Surg. 2001;108:2160 -2161.

Hacker DC, Freeman JL. Intracranial extension of a nasal dermoid cyst in a 56-year-old man. Head Neck 1994;16:366- 71.

Harley, E. H., and Erdman, J. P. Dorsal nasal cyst formation. Arch. Otolaryngol. Head Neck Surg. 116: 105, 1990

Imholte M, Schwartz HC. Respiratory implantation cyst of the mandible after chin augmentation: report of case. Otolaryngol— Head Neck Surg 2001;124:586–7.

Inchingolo F, Tatullo M, Abenavoli FM, Marrelli M, Inchingolo AD, Servili A, Inchingolo AM, Dipalma G. (2010). A hypothetical correlation between hyaluronic acid gel and development of cutaneous metaplastic synovial cyst. Head Face Med. 15, 6:13.

Johnson CM, Anderson JR. The deviated nose- its correction. Laryngoscope 1977;87,1680-4

Karapantzos I, Behrmann R, Simaskos N. Paranasal mucous cyst: a rare finding following septorhinoplasty. Rhinology 1999;37:190–1.

Koeller KK, Alamo L, Adair CF and Smirniotopoulos JG. (1999). Congenital Cystic Masses of the Neck: Radiologic-Pathologic Correlation. Radiographics, 19, pp. 121-146.

Kotzur A., Gubisch W. Mucous cyst--a postrhinoplasty complication: outcome and prevention. Plast Reconstr Surg. 1997 Aug;100(2):520-4.

Lawson W, Kessler S, Biller HF (1983) Unusual and fatal complications of rhinoplasty. Arch Otolaryngol Head Neck Surg 109:164–169

Leong AC, Sharp HR. (2009). Nasal septal cyst: a rare phenomenon. Auris Nasus Larynx. 36, 1, pp. 96-9.

Liu ES, Kridel RW. (2003). Postrhinoplasty nasal cysts and the use of petroleumbased ointments and nasal packing. Plast Reconstr Surg, 112, pp. 282–287.

McGregor, M. W., O'Connor, G. B., and Saffier, S. Complications of rhinoplasty: I. Skin and subcutaneous tissues. J. Int. Coll. Surg. 30: 179, 1958.

Mouly R. Le kyste mucoide, complication inhabtuelle de la rhinoplastie. Ann Chir Plast 1970;15:153–5.

Ntomouchtsis A, Kechagias N, Xirou P, Triaridis A, Xinou K, Vahtsevanos K. Recurrent glabellar mucous cyst: a rare postrhinoplasty complication.Oral Maxillofac Surg. 2010 Jun;14(2):129-32.

Pausch NC, Bertolini J, Hemprich A, Hierl T. Inclusion mucous cysts of the nose: a late complication after septorhinoplasty in two cleft lip patients. Cleft Palate Craniofac J. 2010 Nov;47(6):668-72

Raine C, Williamson SLH, McLean NR. Mucous cyst of the alar base: a rare complication following rhinoplasty. Br J Plast Surg 2003;56(2):176–7.

Rees T, ed. The osteocartilaginous vault. In: Aesthetic Plastic Surgery. Philadelphia, Pa: WB. Saunders Co; 1980;114-176

Rettinger G, Zenkel M. Skin and soft tissue complications. Facial Plast Surg. 1997;13:51-9

Riedel F, Bersch C, Hörmann K (2007) Dorsal nasal mass formation—postrhinoplasty cyst. HNO 55:472–47

Rohrich RJ, Krueger JK, Adams WP, Hollier LH. Achieving consistency in the lateral nasal osteotomy during rginoplasty: An external perforated technique. *Plast. Reconstr. Surg.* 108: 2122, 2001

Rohrich RJ, Janis JE, Adams WP, Krueger JK. An update on the lateral nasal osteotomy in rhinoplasty: An anatomic endoscopic comparison of the external versus the internal approach. *Plast. Reconstr. Surg.* 111: 2461, 2003.

Romo T 3rd, Rizk SS, Suh GD (1999) Mucous cyst formation after rhinoplasty. Arch Facial Plast Surg 1: 208–211

Senechal G, Senechal B, Mamelle G (1981) Une complication rare e tardive des rhinoplasties. Ann Oto-Laryng (Paris) 98:385–386

Shulman Y, Westreich M. Postrhinoplasty mucous cyst of the nose. Plast Reconstr Surg 1983;71:421–2.

Struijs B, Bauwens LJ.Post-rhinoplasty mucous cyst formation of the nasal dorsum. B-ENT. 2010;6(4):295-8.

Tan Ergin N., Akkuzu B. Mucous cyst of the nasal dorsum. Rhinology 2000;38,206-7

Tardy ME. Rhinoplasty, In: Tardy ME, Kastenbauer ER. Head and Neck Surgery. Thieme, 1995,pp239-302

Tastan E, Kavuzlu A, Demirci M, Sungu N. A unique case of a postrhinoplasty epidermoid cyst. Rhinology 2010;48,244-6

Toriumi DM, Johnson CM (1990) Revision rhinoplasty: case study. In: Toriumi DM, Johnson CM (eds) Open structure rhinoplasty. WB Saunders, Philadelphia, PA, pp 464–469

Zerris VA, Annino D, Heilman CB. Nasofrontal dermoid sinus cyst: report of two cases. Neurosurgery 2002;51:811- 4.

Zijlker TD, Vuyk HD. Nasal dorsal cyst after rhinoplasty. Rhinology. 1993; 31:89 –91.